I0423084

NUTRITION MYSTERY SOLVED

Praise for *Nutrition Mystery Solved*

There has not been a topic more studied, controversial and misunderstood by practicing physicians and other health care professionals than diet and nutrition. As an interventional cardiologist I have observed firsthand the nefarious results of the "Western" diets on human and even animal health. I was also struck by the obvious lack of health benefits of the commonly recommended dietary interventions promoted by nutritionists, dietitians, health gurus and the like.

Driven by a strong desire to live a long and healthy life, Mr. Mamonov has spent decades painstakingly researching this fascinating topic. He presents evidence based data from a historic comparative perspective. What sets him aside from other authors is his truly holistic approach. The presentation of various other factors and interventions related to energy and metabolism that should promote longevity renders the lecture captivating and thought provoking.

In an age where access to information is more readily accessible than ever, where education has moved out of the classical class room, Mr. Mamonov's chapter on diet and nutrition is an excellent review and could be easily included in any medical school curriculum.

Velisar Rill, M.D.

It's hard for me to calculate how many tens of thousands, perhaps millions, of lives will be saved by this Chapter 15 (previous title of the book). I sincerely knew that after reading only 30 pages. Now that I've read it thoroughly, a couple of times, I'm so grateful you are such a careful and meticulous scientist, in the manner of Dr. Bjorn Nordenstrom at the Karolinska Institut in Sweden, who was the head of the Nobel Committee for 15 years and who carefully and solitarily did his own research until he found an internationally used cure for cancer.

Because you may have saved my life and my family's and my patients' lives with your book that scrutinizes incomplete research, faulty conclusions, and cherry picking of so-called 'experts' who wanted to prove a point, but who were not aware of the whole picture and of exciting international studies that contradict accepted 'truths' in the U.S. that have caused accelerated disease and death here. Thank you for being you. Your mother in heaven is so proud of you.

Dr. Ann Wigmore's Dr. Flora

The true eureka moment came when I got hold of Dr. Mamonov's "Nutrition Mystery Solved: Why Japanese Researchers Would Never Eat Fried Food." His brave and bold approach to questioning as well as backing up with scientific data completely shattered all the myths about fats and oil. This book elaborates in minute detail and with out of the box thinking. After finishing reading the book I felt as if I've attained nutritional enlightenment and have been liberated. I stopped deep frying altogether to protect my body and soul. His no-nonsense approach is a personal health blessing in my life. This book is a must read!

Puvaneswari P. M., M.B.A.

A detailed, scientific and personal account/treatise/exposition based on Mamonov's 2001 book, "Control for Life Extension." This current book was written partly to bring clarity to less substantiated claims of many popular directions, health policies and practices. This book conflicts with "conventional wisdom" when navigating health issues.

He brings information, cites studies, and reveals stories of his personal experiences to apply and test his ideas on health. This book is a **Gift** to straighten crossed-eyed views, shallow thinking and wide-☐ spread fads on the subject. This expansive presentation "connects more dots." This manifesto is a foundation for scientific expansion. This gift of thought research was not paid for by grants or foundations. This book may inspire others to contribute their best to our world.

Question the motivation of the researcher... follow the money!

N. Jacob

~

A book that goes beyond recommendations on food for a healthy life. A compilation of and reference to many scientific studies makes for a better understanding of such a complex issue. A great and overdue work!

Much of my life spent in many countries, particular in Africa, made me aware that people with access to a limited variety of food resources intuitively make choices of best tolerated products, but not so when they are exposed to the variety of industrial food products of our modern civilization. A summary of the findings of this study in the introduction would make for improved reading.

Eugene Boelens, A former Official of the United Nations
Development Programme.

NUTRITION MYSTERY SOLVED

WHY JAPANESE RESEARCHERS WOULD NEVER EAT FRIED FOOD

Valery Mamonov, Ph.D.

Amazon KDP Publishing

This publication contains the opinions and ideas of it's author. It is sold with the understanding that the author and publisher are not engaged in rendering health services in the book. The reader should consult his or her own medical and health providers as appropriate before adopting any of the suggestions in this book or drawing inferences from it.

The author and publisher specifically disclaim all responsibility for any liability, loss or risk, personal or otherwise, which is incurred as a consequence, directly or indirectly, of the use and application of any of the contents of this book.

Copyright © 2020 by Valery Mamonov

All rights reserved. No part of this book may be used or reproduced in any manner whatsoever without written permission from the publisher except in the case of brief quotations embodied in critical articles and reviews.

First Amazon KDP Publishing trade paperback edition December 2019

Cover design by Susan E. Smith
Manufactured in the United States of America

10 9 8 7 6 5 4 3 2 1

Mamonov, Valery, 1941–
Nutrition Mystery Solved: Why Japanese Researchers Would Never Eat Fried Food / Valery Mamonov
        pages   cm
1. Fats in human nutrition. 2. Carbohydrates in human nutrition.
3. Proteins in human nutrition. II. Title. [1. Self-help. 2.
Health. –Popular works.]
Includes references, glossary, and index.
    RA776.75.M263 613'.0438 909-920

This book is dedicated to
my mother, Anna Danilovna,
guardian
throughout my life,
who continues
to guide me
from heaven
even still.

CONTENTS

Acknowledgments.. x

Introduction... xii

1. Foundations of Health..1
2. Blood Type A1 Diet...5
3. Good Fats, Bad Fats...13
4. Lipid Peroxidation..23
5. Animal Fat Will Not Kill You But Low Cholesterol Will.......33
6. Is Omega-3 Healthy?..42
7. Saturated Fat..47
8. Stability of Saturated Fat......................................57
9. Trans Fats...64
10. Fats in Health and Disease....................................78
11. How Essential Are Carbohydrates?............................93
12. Deleterious Effects of Carbohydrates........................105
13. Proteins...111
14. How Much Protein Do We Need?...............................117
15. Excessive Protein Consumption and Cancer..................122
16. Conclusion..125

Appendix 1..128

Glossary..132

References..141

Index...166

About the Author..175

ACKNOWLEDGMENTS

Many people have helped me acquire healthy habits and become health-conscious which was not the case until I was 37. I am forever indebted to my Russian yoga teachers, Vladimir Samol and Eugene Bazh, from whom I learned various diets, exercises, meditation, body-cleansing methods, and the mind-body connection. They continue to guide me from the other side and I want to express to them my abundant gratitude. I must also give special thanks to Dr. Ray Peat, PhD and Dr. Joel D. Wallach, D.M.V., N.D. whose ideas on the detriments to health of polyunsaturated fatty acids (PUFAs) and grain products have inspired my research.

I express my utmost gratitude to my editors and dear friends, Norman Emanuel and Dr. Flora van Orden. Norman spent endless hours painstakingly correcting my manuscript and making it readable and understandable. Dr. Flora greatly contributed to editing as well and suggested that Chapter 15 on nutrition and diets, which is an upgrade of a similar chapter in my previous book, "Control for Life Extension. A Personalized Holistic Approach," could be published as a separate book. Lately, Dr. Flora suggested a different book title, "Nutrition Mystery Solved: Why Japanese Researchers Would Never Eat Fried Food." Drs. C. Norm Shealy, M.D., Ph.D., Dr. Flora, Velisar Rill,

M.D., and Puvaneswari "Vennes" P. M., MBA spent a lot of their time in reading my manuscript and gave me wonderful endorsements. I am so thankful to them too.

A part of my research in this book is devoted to the heart disease and latitude connection from which I learned how deleterious to my health was living in the state of Maine for 20 years. Maine is reputed to be a "nice and cold" state. Although I lived in Russia in cold areas and was used to a cold climate when I was younger, to me, Maine winters became increasingly cold as I grew older. In the depth of the winter, my hands would become frigid and circulation in them would be impaired.

Eventually I moved to Florida and I give my special thanks to my friends Boris Klovsky, Valery and Jacob Barvashov, Walter Eizenberg, my daughter Victoria and her husband Stephen Mourousas and Kaori Yamane who aided me in my relocation. Nancy Jacob, my dear friend in Maine for 20 years, helped me move with my belongings to Florida, to find my new residence, and encouraged me with her laughs at my jokes while she was reading the manuscript.

I want also to thank my dear friends Vladimir and Slava Ostrov, who helped me to emigrate from Russia. They always encouraged me in my writings, provided me with their wise advice, and took my circumstances close to their hearts.

I would like to express my heartfelt thanks to S.E. Smith, the New York Times/USA TODAY Bestselling author, for her guidance and expertise navigating the labyrinth of publishing. My thanks go also to Laurelle Santamaria for her help formatting the book.

I apologize to any I have neglected to mention also worthy of my praise and thanks. This is not due to my lack of gratitude to them, but rather because of my failures of memory.

INTRODUCTION

This book on nutrition and diets is an upgraded and modified version of Chapter 15 in my previous book, "Control for Life Extension. A Personalized Holistic Approach." While doing research for upgrading it I became interested in some related health issues such as heart disease and cancer as related to food and they are discussed herein. A big part of the book is focused on fats because they became and still remain the most misunderstood part of our nutrition.

When I arrived in the USA in 1996, to my surprise, I found America was in the state of war with fats. A whole generation or two have been brainwashed with propaganda and "health" advice, which continues to this day, the presumed benefit being the reduction of fat consumption. Because of my different background, I remained unbiased and fats for me have always been and remain just one of the three macronutrients, the other two being proteins and carbohydrates.

Of all different types of fats, saturated fat is considered by "health authorities" to be bad for us and polyunsaturated fatty acids (PUFAs) in vegetable oils good and even "heart-healthy." Just to the contrary, based on solid research, it is shown herein that the healthiest are coconut oil, butter and beef fat that have the highest saturated fat content and the most deleterious to health are PUFAs in vegetable oils. This is crucial, especially with the recent popularity of the keto-genic diet (80% fat) for weight loss and other health issues, to know which fats are beneficial and which are not.

There is, however, a kind of fat, which has deleterious effects to human health, that both official policy makers and their critics agree upon: *trans* fats. *Trans* fats are created in the process of hydrogenation as well as during deodorization, refining, and deep frying in vegetable oils, which is carried out at high temperatures ranging from 320°F (180°C) to 464°F (270°C). After 70 years of research, the FDA banned *trans* fats in the United States on June 16, 2015, giving food producers three years to comply. Although food producers claim 0% *trans* fats on food labels, if analyzed, they can be found in foods deep-fried in vegetable oils. It is another reason to avoid vegetable oils of any sort. The *trans* fats issue is discussed in detail in the book.

Fats can have the opposite effect in health and disease, and this issue is poorly understood. For instance, omega 3 fatty acids with their three double bonds, which are subject to oxidative damage, can be harmful to a healthy person and in one study they even were called a "cancer initiator." On the flip side, they are so toxic that they can kill cancer cells in a person so stricken (flaxseed oil rich in omega-3 in the Johanna Budwig protocol). The same, although to a lesser degree, holds for omega-6, which was called a "cancer promoter." This matter will also be discussed.

The issue of healthy fats is very important for the overall health of Blood type A1 people which I am also. In the USA, they comprise 33.6% of the population or one in three people. Their average life expectancy is the shortest, only sixty-two years, a full quarter of a century shorter than that of blood type Os. They are the most vulner-able of all Blood types and heart disease, stroke, cancer, and diabetes kill Blood type A1s prematurely.

I devised a blood type A1 diet which I have adhered to for the last five years. I believe that this diet has sustained me in that I am still alive and free from medications at my age of 79. Also, I am tall, my height is 6' 2". As studies show, if we are taller than 5'11", for each additional inch we need to subtract 2 years from our average life expectancy. In my case it is 6 years. Sixty-two minus six is fifty-six, and it means that I am supposed to have expired twenty-two years ago on average. My answer is in a proper diet and a healthy lifestyle.

I also believe that the Blood and constitutional types, other than mine, can benefit from this diet as well. The Blood type A1 diet avoids a few food categories such as legumes, vegetable oils, grain products, and dairy products and seems to be very restricted. In actuality, however, it is quite varied and nutritious, with over 60 food items to choose from.

Vegetable oils, as pro-inflammatory factors leading to endothelium dysfunction of blood vessels, are involved in the clogging up of the coronary arteries, which is deemed to be the main cause of the heart or coronary artery disease (CAD). Lowering blood cholesterol is advised to prevent cardiovascular disease. However, studies show an increased risk of cancer death at low cholesterol levels.

Another constituent of our food, carbohydrates, may bring about deleterious effects to our system. Our body responses to carbohydrates by the secretion of hormones (growth factors) such as insulin and insulin like growth factors IGF 1 and IGF 2. These growth factors including insulin prompt our cells to grow and proliferate which can be dangerous if the new cells are cancerous.

Sugars derived from carbohydrates when high temperatures are used in cooking react with amino acids binding to them and thus impairing their normal function. It creates advanced glycation end products (AGE) in which the protein molecules are stiffened and degraded in an irreversible way.

Carbohydrates taken in excess can cause a disorder called *lipemia,* or "fatty blood." The concentration of triglycerides in the blood is increased through the process of *de novo* lipogenesis in which the liver creates fats from glucose. The proponents of the low fat, plant-based diet erroneously accuse animal fat and cholesterol of causing *lipemia,* thus base their movement's philosophy on a false premise.

Unlike the two other basic macronutrients in food, fats and carbo-☐ hydrates, used by our bodies as sources of energy, proteins serve as a building material as well. Each and every body part, organ or tissue is composed of proteins. They also are an essential part of connective tissue, blood, lymph, hormones, enzymes, blood cells, and antibodies. Proteins must be broken down into amino acids by our digestive system so that cells can assimilate them.

Nine of 21 amino acids needed to maintain health cannot be synthesized by our body. They are known as essential amino acids and have to be obtained from food. Not all essential amino acids are beneficial to our health. Tryptophan, methionine and cysteine high in muscle meats are considered "problem" amino acids. Tryptophan was found to be carcinogenic and restriction of these three amino acids resulted in an increased life span in rodents. As compared with muscle meats, gelatin contains only small amounts of cysteine, methionine, and histidine and can serve as a main source of protein. Good sources of gelatin are meat stock and bone broth made from oxtail or beef legs.

The protein amount in the proposed Blood type A1 diet is close to the Optimal Diet developed by Jan Kwasniewski, MD of Poland. For a 5'11" (180 cm) individual, protein requirements would equal 64 grams (2.25 oz). Excessive protein consumption is associated with different kinds of cancer and countries with high protein consumption have higher death rates from cancer. Temperance and moderation, the motto of long-lived people and centenarians, once again holds sway.

1

FOUNDATIONS OF HEALTH

Should you ask me what's best to eat,
I'll tell you: eat right for your type, you should
Eat yams with butter, honey, eggs and meat,
And don't stuff your face with food.

L etting philosophers argue about the old question—that is, whether reality is of the nature of thought (mind over matter) or whether all phenomena, including those of the mind, are due to material agencies (matter over mind)—we will go straight to our objective: in achieving longevity, both body and mind must be equally healthy. It is a widely accepted hypothesis in biology that a human is "...not mind and body, but body and mind in one. Body is one aspect of this unity, mind is another," said H.G. Wells, et al., in their book *The Science of Life* [1]. "Man, in this hypothesis, is not Mind plus Body; he is a Mind-Body," they added. It is only for convenience that we distinguish between body, mind, and spirit, and separately study physiological and psychological aspects of the unity, which is a single universal human being.

Which constituents are essential for a healthy and sound body, mind, and spirit? Both Western and Oriental thought share similar ideas in this respect. The famous Greek physician Hippocrates (c. 460 – c. 377 BC), the father of Western medicine, taught that good health can be attained and maintained only through the proper balance of physical, mental, and spiritual energies. It was natural for him and other ancient physicians to acknowledge the importance of a *holistic* approach, which incorporates body, mind and soul.

According to Leon Chaitow [2] of London, England, positive health depends on three factors, which are interconnected. The first of these is the body's structural system, including all the muscles, bones, ligaments, nerves, blood vessels, organs, and their functions. The second factor is the body's biochemical processes, which involve the absorption and utilization of nutrients, and the elimination of wastes, along with the complicated biochemical relationships that are the key to cellular function and health. The third factor consists of the mind and emotions, as well as the spiritual dimension of each person.

The modern Oriental approach to good health and longevity holds that body, mind, and spirit have to be well balanced and in good harmony with nature. "Food, drink, emotions, stress, and what we think add to the body chemistry and make us who we are. We are a combination of our family genes and environment," say Shizuko Yamamoto and Patrick McCarty in their book, *Whole Health Shiatsu*. "You may want to carefully observe how you think, breathe, eat, move, sleep, and maintain relationships, for these are the six fundamentals of health" [3, p.42] they add.

Everybody eats—eating is a part of everyone's life. Everybody needs food to live. Food gives us life, and food is life itself. All living creatures need food. Air and sunlight are food for plants. Plants are food for animals. Plants and animals are food for humans. It wouldn't be an exaggeration to say that food is absolutely necessary for our survival and health. Ordinary people in ordinary conditions can't live without food.

There are cases in the history of mankind and even today in which people abstained from food for years and even decades. However, these few people achieved special spiritual states that are unattainable for most people. Modern science still fails to explain the phenomenon of surviving long term without food and being alive and healthy. I believe that we will have many discoveries in this field in the future.

A deep understanding that food and health are closely interrelated is one of the fundamental ideas of ancient medical systems, such as the Indian Ayurveda and Traditional Chinese Medicine. Ayurveda has taught for thousands of years that our health is largely determined by what we eat. The Yellow Emperor of China (2698- 2589 BC) is known for his appreciation of the idea that a balanced diet is absolutely essential for maintaining one's health and avoiding illnesses. Modern scientific research, especially nutritional discoveries of the last two decades, gave credit to many kinds of healing foods that can improve our health, sometimes even better than drugs.

Plants use the energy of the sun to combine substances from the soil and air to produce complex substances that make up living matter. We are not able to do that and must rely on food by eating plants or the animals that ate plants. According to Western science, food—solid or liquid—functions for our body primarily in two ways, nutritional and energetic, as follows:

• Food provides substances needed to build and renew our cells, bones, muscles, and tissues, and for our growth, maintenance, repair, and reproduction.

• As a fuel, food produces body heat and energy necessary for performing physical and mental work.

These two functions are fulfilled by the substances in food called *nutrients*, which are divided into the following two major types:

• macronutrients (proteins, carbohydrates, and fats) that contain calories

• micronutrients (vitamins and minerals) that have no caloric value

To maintain good health, all these nutrients (a total of fifty [4, p.231] to ninety [5, p.133]) must be supplied to the body in sufficient quantities, fine quality, and proper proportions. Nutrients have existed in food since the beginning of time, but scientists discovered them only within the last hundred years or so. Sometimes four more vital substances–water, fiber, oxygen, and light–are considered nutrients; however, fiber (insoluble) is composed mostly of cellulose (complex carbohydrates) that goes through the digestive tract undigested. "Nearly all indigestible plant fiber is cellulose—wood being the most striking example" [6, p.42].

Water as a nutrient is overshadowed by the food we eat, but it comes to light under certain circumstances: fasting with water can last up to ninety days [7], but dry fasting can last only about eighteen days [8]. Oxygen and sunlight are essential for all vital processes in the body. Nutrition is the way our body assimilates and utilizes food for its development, maintenance, and repair.

Oriental medicine has a somewhat different approach to food—it holds that solid, liquid, particle, and vibration forms of food are essential to our body. Although solid, liquid (macronutrients), and particle (minerals and vitamins) forms of food are all the same, it is the vibration food that contrasts with the Western approach. Vibration foods are sunshine, weather, cosmic radiation, smell, prana, magnetic fields, and even the rotation of the earth. All life on earth is dependent on these powerful vibrations.

Air that contains nitrogen, oxygen, and carbon dioxide must also be considered as a source of food for our body. There are many types of food for the mind as well: thoughts, dreams, meditation, study, investigation, research, creation, watching movies and TV, listening to music and the radio, conversations with others, one's internal dialogue, fantasies, and many others are examples of food for the mind.

Everything around us feeds our five senses too. Sensitive people can feel the emanations from places, objects, things, and people; some may call it extra-sensory perception (ESP) [9]. The phenomenon that plants have the ESP capabilities was experimentally proved [10, p.105]. Again, I am trying to show the full range of all possible kinds of food. You may think that I am exaggerating when I talk about smell or prana as a kind of food; probably you would be right, but who knows?

2

BLOOD TYPE A1 DIET

For as he eats & drinks he grows
Younger & younger every day; …
—William Blake, *The Mental Traveler*

If I am to propose a diet suitable for both my Blood type A1 and to promote health and longevity, it will be as follows. In this diet I avoid whole categories of food, each for a specific reason, that I believe is harmful to you and me.

Foods in the Blood type A1 diet:

1. have minimized blood clotting lectins [11, p.23-8; 12, p.203-4],

2. are low in polyunsaturated fatty acids PUFAs.

The higher PUFA content, the greater is the peroxide value, a measure of lipid per-oxidation, which makes oils rancid, stale, and toxic [13, 14].

3. are void of grain products, which are high in lectins [12, p.203-4] and PUFAs.

Of all grains, I eat only white rice, which has the lowest PUFA content (0.2%) and helps me to maintain my weight. With my Mesomorphic Ectomorph constitution and increased metabolism, I easily lose weight and have difficulty gaining it back—an issue that is just the opposite of most people.

4. contain no beans, peas or lentils.

Legumes are high in lectins [12, p.203-4], contain glucosinolates, which inhibit thyroid gland function [15].

5. are low in nightshades (potatoes, tomatoes, eggplant, bell peppers, and tobacco).

Nightshades are pro-inflammatory and pro-arthritic foods [16].

The only exclusion for me is potatoes, which were a staple of my ancestors in Russia and seem to be tolerable to me. I eat about 3 oz of potatoes a day, in my mushroom soup, and not every day. On some days, I alternate them with sweet potatoes and yams. At 78, I do not have arthritis. When I sell my book at farmers' markets, among other signs I display is a "Free Arthritis Test" sign. People ask what it is and I have them bend their fingers, by putting fingernails against finger-nails, and pressing their palms together to close the gap between them, so their palms touch each other. I show them how I do it (Pictures 15-1 and 15-2).

Surprisingly, many people even some teenagers fail to pass the test because they eat pro-arthritic foods, notably, nightshades, foods deep fried in vegetable oils that are loaded with *trans* fats, processed foods and sugary drinks. Then I say, "I am sorry, I am 78 and do not have arthritis, also I don't wear glasses, have no hearing aids, and do not wear diapers." The last one usually makes them laugh and, on that happy note, they leave my table without buying my book.

6. contain no cruciferous (cabbage family) vegetables.

Cruciferous vegetables are goitrogenic and suppress thyroid gland function [17]. Again, there is an exclusion for sauerkraut, which my Russian parents preserved and ate in the winter time and I eat it too. Sauerkraut is a rich source of Vitamin C, probiotics, and other vital nutrients [18].

7. free from nuts or seeds, which are high in lectins [11, p.203-4] and PUFAs [12, 13].

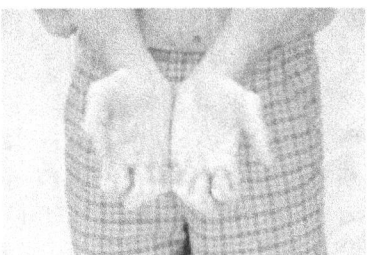

Picture 15-1. Actively Bent Fingers

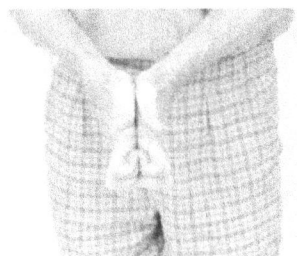

Picture 15-2. Palms Pressed Against Each Other

8. void of vegetable oils or their butters, such as peanut, almond, cashews, and other butters that also are high in lectins [11, p.203-4] and PUFAs [12, 13].

Of all nuts and vegetable oils, I eat only coconuts, coconut and macadamia nut oils, which are very low in PUFAs and high in stable saturated fats. Macadamia nuts that are sold in the health food stores in this country are very expensive, around $20 a pound, and I usually don't bother buying them. Instead, while in Maine, I would buy macadamia nut oil, for $15 a one pint bottle and use it about 1 Tbsp a day for my salads.

After my cruise ship trip from Los Angeles to Australia in 2014, I stayed for another two weeks in the Sydney area and found that most food items in the grocery stores were at least twice as expensive as in the USA. Some items like ginger and garlic were five to seven times more expensive. The only item that was half the price was macadamia nut oil because they grow them there.

9. are lacking dairy products.

Blood type As and Os have antibodies against galactose, a terminal sugar in Blood type B antigens and dairy products alike and our immune system attacks them as it does in the case of an improper blood transfusion [10, p.151]. Because of that reason, dairy products are suitable for Blood type Bs only and, to some extent, to Blood type ABs.

10. are void of soy products.

Soy products are high in lectins [11, p.203-4], allergens, anti-nutrients, and toxins [19].

11. contain no poultry or pork.

These meats are high in PUFAs [12, 13]. Chickens, turkey and pigs are monogastric (one stomach) animals [20], which readily transfer PUFAs into their eggs, tissues and fats from their feed, based in this country, on corn and soy beans that are high in polyunsaturated fats PUFAs. For instance, in 100 g of yellow corn, which contains 4.7 g of total fat, PUFA comprises 2.2 g or 46.8% [21]. In 100 g of soy flour, total fat is 20.6 g of which PUFA is 11.7 g or 56.8% [22].

If corn and soy is fed to polygastric (many stomachs) animals, also called ruminants [20], then PUFAs are metabolized in their stomachs by the process of hydrolysis and bio-hydrogenation with the help of bacteria and much less of PUFAs go into their meat, fat, and milk [23].

Although my diet seems to be very restricted, in actuality it is quite nutritious and varied. It includes 61 food items to choose from and is balanced in its macro and micronutrient content of raw and cooked items. This is a quite palatable diet of lamb, beef, butter, seaweed, crab meat, caviar, honey, coconut oil, etc. that has sustained me quite pleas-☐ antly for the last five years, and it is not extreme. It contains 12% carbohydrates, 74% fat, and 10% protein. I take some supplements too.

Also, I do not advocate a fanatic adherence to my fare and I believe that occasional deviation will not do much harm. If a Holy Communion offered in the church was made from wheat, it is too small an amount to worry about. I occasionally eat some goat or Swiss cheese, seemingly without adverse effects. In the case of mini doses of poisons that we encounter, the "nutritional hormesis" concept comes into play [24]. It states that a small amount of toxin is even beneficial to our systems. Vladimir Samol, my yogi friend, used to say, "You know, 'father,' the elephants in Africa sometimes chew on a little toxic grass to poison themselves down, otherwise, they would 'explode of internal over-vitality.'"

Food items of the Blood type A1 diet, its nutritional value, and shopping list are displayed in Appendix 1.

In its macronutrient content, the Blood type A1 diet is close to the Optimal Diet developed by Jan Kwasniewski, MD of Poland. His high-fat (80%), low-carbohydrate (4%), and optimal protein (12%) diet proved its effectiveness by dramatic improvements and even cures of "various illnesses as Buerger's disease, arthritis, Gastrointestinal disor-☐ der, obesity, diabetes and many others" [26]. However, Kwasniewski's diet heavily depends on eggs, pork, and lard and despite of his success in Poland and other countries, it can not be applied in this country because the feed of chickens and pigs is very different.

In main-land America, the PUFA content in the lard of pigs (fed with corn and soybeans) is 32% and in the Caribbean countries where their feed is coconuts, low-fat fish and sweet potatoes – 3% [27] or 11 times less. The proposed diet contains just a mere 2% of PUFAs. Its main source of animal protein is lamb or beef.

According to Kwasniewski, the ideal proportion between protein, fat and carbohydrates in the diet is "from 1:2.5:0.5 to 1:3.5:0.5 meaning that with every gram of protein 2.5 to 3.5 grams of fat and half a gram of carbohydrates should be eaten" [26]. It makes the optimal nutrition regimen a high fat, low carbohydrate diet.

The **optimal amount of protein** in grams is determined as 80% of the person's **ideal weight** (measured in kilograms), which is equal to their height in cm minus 100. For a 5'11" (180 cm) individual, the ideal weight would be 80 kg (176 lb) and protein requirements would equal 64 grams (2.25 oz). Depending on the person's weight, the protein intake may fluctuate by plus or minus 10% [26].

It perfectly corresponds with the dietary advice of the US Institute of Medicine of the National Academies (IOM), which recommends that the "average person should consume 0.8 g/per kilogram of body weight, or 0.36 g/lb, of protein per day" [28].

Kwasniewski' diet is called the "Polish Atkins Diet" because of their similarity in low carbohydrates. However, Kwasniewski's diet contains less protein than Atkins' diet. For comparison, the recommen-☐ ded protein intake for a 5'11" man on the Atkins diet is 19 oz (133g) [29, p.43] or twice as much.

Excessive protein consumption has a few negative effects. It can cause gout because of the high purines content in meats and may "worsen kidney function in people with kidney disease" [30]. High protein foods such as beef, fish, eggs, and yogurt impose an increased insulin demand on the pancreas [31]. Also, Blood type A1 people have low secretions of hydrochloric acid [11, p.98], which can result in putrefaction of poorly digested animal foods, cause osteoporosis due to altered calcium and other minerals metabolism, and a whole host of different ailments. "A long list of diseases frequently associated with low stomach acidity includes: diabetes mellitus, both underactive and overactive thyroid, childhood asthma, eczema, gallbladder disease, osteoporosis, rheumatoid arthritis, chronic hives, lupus erythematosus, weak adrenals, chronic hepatitis, vitiligo, and rosacea" [32, p.33].

With its 74% fat content, the Blood type A1 diet is less ketogenic [33] than the Kwasniewski's diet (80% fat), and hence might be more sustainable in the long run. The study of sustainability of the Kwas-☐ niewski diet did not find any long-term (>1 year) deleterious effects [34]. However, a severe (to 4%) restriction of carbohydrates that are a primary source of energy for the body might make it difficult to stick to it, say, for a few years.

Both the Blood type A1 and Kwasniewski's diets are similar in avoiding whole categories of food, notably, grains, pasta, flours, starches, peas & beans, and skim milk, and emphasizing animal fats, meats, giblets, and meat stock/bone broth. There are distinctions, though, e.g., cheese, whole milk, cream, seeds, nuts, and vegetable oils (limited to 1-2%) that are allowed in the Kwasniewski's diet but are foods to avoid in the Blood type A1 diet.

Blood type Os, with their increased secretion of hydrochloric acid, have an advantage over Blood type As, which lack hydrochloric acid [35, 36, p.20]. Blood type A's can enhance their system to produce stomach acid to overcome indigestion with carminative (stomach soothing) herbs such as camomile, peppermint, bay leaves, ginseng, goldenseal, angelica, ginger, marjoram, coriander, rosemary, red pepper, and dozens of other herbs in teas and tinctures [37, p.275-77; 38, p.353-54]. Of the animal origin, raw hog stomach [39] and raw liver, if supplemented to the diet, could be beneficial in improving stomach function [32, p.35]. The hog's stomach extract, Ventriculin, given to five patients with chronic atrophic gastritis (supplementing their diets with doses averaging 30-60 grams per day) resulted in marked symptomatic improvement in all of them [40].

In Russian folk medicine, the desiccated inner lining of the chicken stomach called cuticula (epidermis, a yellow film, bitter in taste), dried and made into a powder is used to increase the production of stomach acid [41]. If you buy gizzards in the supermarket in this country, they are already processed and the lining is always absent.

Regarding low stomach acid prevalent in Blood type A1s, a few years ago while in Maine, I asked a farmer to sell me unprocessed chicken stomachs with the cuticula (inner lining) intact in them. She slaughtered 20 chickens and sold me their stomachs. I took the linings off, freeze- and then room temperature dried them, ground in coffee mill, and have used 1/8 tsp after meat-containing meals. I do the same now after I have moved to Florida. This helps me to produce more hydrochloric acid and, therefore, to improve my digestion. The only hope for my blood group A1 with its increased risk of cancer is a healthy lifestyle, being the crux of my book.

The intrinsically weak stomach acid in Blood type A people causes both indigestion and malabsorption [32]. One more way to increase the strength of stomach acid is to take betaine hydrochloride supplements [32, p.35]. However, a much better way is to stimulate our system to produce it. Animal foods such as meat, fish, and eggs require strong hydrochloric acid to be broken down and digested. When we eat these foods, we train our body to produce more of it.

The Blood type A1 diet provides a necessary amount of animal protein that encourages our system to produce hydrochloric acid. That ensures a proper metabolism, which in turn helps to avoid conditions like arthritis, osteoporosis, hepatitis, and others [32]. For people with liver disease such as hepatitis, Dr. Ray Peat warns against alcohol and advocates fructose and saturated fats [42] that are abundant in the Blood type A1 diet.

3

GOOD FATS, BAD FATS

The only way to keep your health is to eat what you don't want, drink what you don't like, and do what you'd rather not.
— Mark Twain

The main fats in the Kwasniewski's diet are animal fats such as lard, bacon fat, beef tallow, butter, and whole fat milk and cream. The only vegetable oil in his diet is olive oil used in his coleslaw and tomato with onions salads [26]. In a comment on the sustainability study of his diet [33] he revealed his attitude to the vegetable oils, saying, "So the heavy emphasis on saturated fats is missed by the paper. A pity, anyone might be left thinking corn oil is a human food..." [34].

The Atkins' diet, in a similar manner, encourages intake of butter, lard, tallow (beef fat), coconut and palm oils, however, by contrast, permits vegetable oils, although warns against overuse of them. "POLYUNSATURATED FATS. Found in vegetable oils such as canola, safflower, grape seed, and flaxseed oils, as well as in fish, polys can be just as beneficial as monounsaturated fats. But use vegetable oils sparingly and carefully" [43, p.56]. "Olive oil is particularly valu-able. All other vegetable oils are allowed, the best being canola, walnut, soybean, grape seed, sesame, sunflower and safflower oils, especially if they are labeled "cold-pressed" or "expeller-pressed" [44, p.127].

As far as canola and other vegetable oils are concerned, Atkins is not alone allowing them in the diet. Many longevity experts do the same.

Dr. Maoshing Ni in his book, *Secrets of Longevity*, teaching us hundreds of ways to live to be 100, asserts, "Monounsaturated fats such as olive oil, sesame oil, canola oil, almond oil, flax oil, and fish oil are good fats" and condemns saturated fats, "The bad fats are the saturated fats and trans fats produced by deep frying: butter, palm kernel oil, peanut oil, coconut oil, and lard" [45, p.31].

Zorba Paster, MD in his book, "The *Longevity Code*," advising us against saturated fats from meat, dairy products, and tropical oils, declares, "On the other hand, unsaturated fats from plant sources, including monounsaturated kind supplied by some nuts and olive or canola oils, may even raise good cholesterol and *lower* bad choles-terol" [46, p.202]. Again, the cholesterol phobia is omnipresent.

Charles B. Inlander & Marie Hodge in their book, *100 Ways to Live to 100,* published in 1992, impart their insights, "Your best bets for cooking are the monounsaturated oils known as canola (rapeseed) and olive oil. The oils to be avoided—those with the most saturated fat— are coconut oil (87 percent) and palm-kernel oil (87 percent)." These authors have more to share, "Saturated oils increase the body's LDL cholesterol (the "bad" kind that contributes to the buildup of fatty plaques in the arteries)" [47, p.23-4].

Interestingly, they mention the case of Verne Gaskins of Milford, Iowa that flies in their own face. Verne "...at age 100, has earned the right to tell the experts they're wrong—at least some of the time! All his life Verne has loved fried foods, bacon and just about anything else nutritionists and doctors consider bad these days. His favorite food: beef. And what about rich, fat-filled ice cream? Every night! [47, p.22]. I have no comments, the adage, "My mind is already made up, don't confuse it with the facts," will do a better job.

Nine years later, Deepak Chopra, MD and David Simon, MD in their book, *Grow Younger, Live Longer*, published in 2001, prescribe, "Your cooking oils should be either monounsaturated, such as olive oil, or polyunsaturated, such as canola, safflower, or sunflower" [48, p.67]. They add, "We do know, based on reliable research, that if you eat an abundance of fresh vegetables, fruits, and whole grains, while reducing your intake of animal fats, you will increase your chances of living healthier and longer" [48, p.63]. You see, they know.

A gerontologist and principal investigator of the New England Centenarian Study, Thomas T. Perls, MD, and co-authors, in their book, *Living to 100*, published in 2001, advocate "Polyunsaturated fats (PF): Found in liquid vegetable oils such as corn (56 percent PF), cottonseed, safflower, soybean, and sunflower (72 percent PF), and also in the fat of fish and nuts (except cashews)" and put into the list to avoid, "Saturated fats: Whole milk, cream, butter, cheese, white bread, meat, poultry skin" and "Cholesterol: Egg yolks, organ meats, tripe, cod liver oil, butter, bacon fat, cream, cheddar cheese" [49, p.184-5].

Among centenarians that Perls studied, "Some ate very little red meat, if any; others ate red meat every day. One of our centenarians had been eating bacon and three eggs every day for breakfast for 15 years."

Dr. Lester Steinberg, 79, the son of a centenarian, explained the eating habits during the formative years of centenarians, "I bet if you really knew what all the centenarians grew up eating, even my mother, you would be astounded. Back at the turn of the century, everyone ate fatty, salty food.... Everyone ate as much sugar and fat as they could find, because it was scarcer" [49, p.59].

Amazingly, Perls, et al., discourage us to eat meat, bacon, and eggs, the very foods that sustained some people to the age of 100. For a real scientist, being politically-correct insures their well-being and promotes longevity.

Yet 25 years later, an epidemiologist, Dr. Martha Clare Morris in her book, *Diet for the Mind*, published in 2017 observes, "Vegetable oils are an important source of what we call healthy fats—that is, monounsaturated and polyunsaturated fats." Also, "When sautéing over medium-high heat, you should use olive, canola, and grape seed oils" [50, p.65-6].

Morris calls red meat, eggs, butter, cheeses and dairy products "brainless food," because they are high in saturated fats. "Butter has a high density of saturated fat: one pat has 4 grams of total fat, of which 2.6 grams (65 percent) is saturated" [50, p.89-93]. Sounds familiar.

If we want to return for a while to the dawn of the cholesterol and saturated fat phobia, we will find, *Dr. Cantor's Longevity Diet*, a book by Alfred J, Cantor, MD., published in 1967. In it we can read, "The polyunsaturated fats are protective to your arteries, and when you reduce the saturated fats in your food and substitute the highly unsaturated fats, you hasten the departure of the cholesterol deposits in your arteries" [51, p.17].

Cantor's recommended edible oils: "Safflower (or corn oil)—three ounces daily," sunflower, soybean, and olive oils and forbidden foods: cheese, butter, lard, whole milk, coconut oil, pork, prepared meats, smoked meats, and delicatessen" [51 p.172-4]. "The Cantor Cocktail" included safflower oil (1 oz), skimmed milk (2 oz), and low calorie soda (3 oz) mixed in the blender [51, p.165]. Sounds palatable, however, all three ingredients are absent in my Blood Type A1 diet.

Of oils recommended on the Dr. Cantor's diet, safflower oil (14.3 % PUFA) is not much higher in PUFA content than olive oil (10.5 %), however, corn oil (54.7 % PUFA) and soybean oil (57.7 % PUFA) are way higher. A daily dose of 3 oz corn oil will result in 46.5 g PUFA intake.

If we assume that Dr. Cantor's diet consisted of 2,500 calories, then PUFA in corn oil alone will comprise 16.8 % of calories, compared with 2 % PUFA in the Blood Type A1 diet, or more than 8 times higher. Apparently, Dr. Cantor was not familiar with the lipid peroxidation issue and the oxidized PUFA-induced free radical damage.

Bradley J. Willcox, MD, D. Craig Willcox, Ph.D., and Makoto Suzuki, MD, the investigators of the Okinawa Centenarian Study, to the contrary, are familiar with lipid peroxidation and even measured lipid peroxides in centenarians and 70-year-old Okinawans. Plasma lipid peroxides of 1.59 units in 100-year-old was found to be nearly two times lower than 2.96 level in the younger population [52, p.63].

Authors want us to live to 100 too and advocate vegetable oils over animal fats. They divide all fats into three categories: "Good" where all vegetable oils, fish, and fish oil are included, "Bad"—all animal fats and tropical oils, and "Ugly"—trans fats such as hydrogenated oils, margarine, fried foods, French fries, cookies, pastries, and pies [52, p.108].

Of course, we must minimize animal food consumption, cut back on red meat, and watch our egg consumption. "The problem with eggs lies in the yolk, which is high in fat and packed with cholesterol" [52, p.134]. Although they acknowledge, "The Okinawan elders use eggs on a regular basis but their portions are small" [52, p.134]. How small, half or a quarter of an egg? Do they eat only whites and do with yolks as what Dr. Cantor did? "I myself like the whites of eggs, and I eat two each morning, throwing away the hard boiled yolks" [51, p.17]. The statement, "When fat circulates in the blood it's called cholesterol" [52, p.113] sounds perplexing to me.

Willcox, et al. mention that Okinawans eat pork, "Less than 10 percent of the elder's diet is meat, mostly pork and poultry" [52 p.73]. Andrew Weil, MD, who wrote foreword to *The Okinawa Program* book and who "made three trips to Okinawa," in his book, *Healthy Aging,* indicates that "They eat a diet quite different from the traditional Japanese diet, with much less salt, more pork, and more tofu, for example" [53, p.33].

My Japanese friends also told me that Okinawans are known in Japan for eating *butaniku* (pork). But the secret is in cooking meat, "When Okinawans eat meat they often stew it for hours (sometimes up to twelve hours), scooping away the fat so that by the time it's ready to eat, the fat content is much lower" [52, p.134]. How much fat is left in the "ready to eat" stewed pork?

What is the fate of that "scooped away" fat, the same as Dr. Cantor's egg yolks—thrown away? I doubt it. Rural folks are not wealthy enough to afford treating food like Dr. Cantor did. They are often religious and would consider it sinful to discard food. Also, they work hard physically burning extra calories, if any, and don't fret over saturated fat and cholesterol as much as doctors do and want us to do. We can clearly see that the *Okinawa Program* doctors take a full leap onto the "vegetable oil is good and animal fat is bad" bandwagon, as, not surprisingly, many other longevity experts do.

We are not done yet reviewing the stances of the longevity experts on vegetable oils and cholesterol. Here are some more. The doctor of pharmacology and gerontologist, Stephen Fulder, Ph.D., in his book, *An End to Aging?* , points out, "Half a nation turned away from butter and cream which is full of cholesterol, to vegetable margarine which is not. Not so many gave up meat. But it is not so simple. Eskimos who eat seal-fat would, according to the cholesterol theory, all be dead by middle age, as would Masai tribesmen with their milk and blood diet. Cholesterol is made by the body, and the high level could be due to manufacture rather than digestion" [54, p.23].

Describing the benefits of ginseng on reducing cholesterol observed in an animal study in Korea, he says, "The level of choles-terol in the blood is related to the production of hardening of the arteries. The amount of cholesterol is both the result of dietary factors and stress-induced changes in body metabolism" [54, p.65]. I believe, Fulder, while moving forward in writing his book from p.23 to p.65, became more politically-correct.

Absolute political correctness (in the war against saturated fat and cholesterol) is the hallmark of the book, *Nutrition in Health and Disease*, by Myron Winick, M.D., published in 1980, which was "designed as a textbook for undergraduate medical students and for students of other health professions and as a practical guide for house staff and practitioners as they deal with patients," who lack "fundamental knowledge of nutrition" [55, p.v].

In the chapter, *Essential Fatty Acid Deficiency*, Winick confines herself to discussing linoleic acid (C18:2ω6) deficiency resulting in dry scaly and flaky skin observed in rats, newborn babies, and adult humans, and growth failure in children. Inclusion in the diet or rubbing olive oil, which contains 9.8 % linoleic acid, are suggested as a means to overcome deficiency [55, p.65].

Interestingly, Winick does not mention at all α-linolenic (from plant sources) or linolenic (from fish or seafood) acid (C18:3ω3), which most nutritional experts regard as an essential (must be obtained from the diet) fatty acid too.

Advocating a "prudent" diet, Winick outlines the dietary guidelines that must be followed: "In general, foods from vegetable sources are more acceptable in the prudent diet than those from animal sources because both saturated fat and cholesterol are more common in foods from animal sources. The greatest concentration of cholesterol is found in eggs and organ meats (fowl eggs, fish roe, beef, calf, or chicken livers, kidneys, heart, and brains)" [55, p.152]. Thank you, Dr. Winick, for listing my favorite foods.

In her push forward of PUFAs, Winick asserts, "The higher the ratio of polyunsaturated to saturated (P : S ratio) the better" [55, p.154]. In the prudent diet, 3 or 4 Tbsp of high PUFA fat should be consumed each day. I believe, medical professionals and their patients would live longer if they could be prudent enough to do just the opposite.

Andrew Weil, MD, in his 2005 book, *Healthy Aging,* displays a less radical view on cholesterol saying, "Until quite recently, the root cause of coronary heart disease was thought to be atherosclerosis, deposits of cholesterol in artery walls as a result of elevated cholesterol levels in the blood. The consensus among cardiologists today is that inflammation of the lining of arteries is more of a root cause. Deposits of cholesterol may even be a flawed healing response of the body, an attempt to patch defects caused by inflammatory damage" [53, p.143].

His disposition on PUFAs is in stark contrast to the above-cited experts: "Minimize the use of polyunsaturated vegetable oils, such as safflower, sunflower, corn, sesame, and soy. They are more likely to oxidize and go rancid than monounsaturated oils like olive and canola" [53, p.149]. Weil seems to favor canola oil saying, "If you want a neutral-tasting oil, use expeller-pressed, organic canola oil" [53, p.248]. Except for canola oil, even organic, it sounds like we a getting closer to the truth.

Further, we can learn from Walter M. Bortz II, MD, a former Co-Chairman of the AMA-ANA Task Force on Aging, who in his 1991 book *We Live Too Short and Die Too Long*, assures that "Cholesterol is good for you. You need it. It contributes greatly to your good functioning, and nearly every tissue in your body has the capacity to make cholesterol from simpler materials" [56, p.238].

Among good things that we get from it is that cholesterol facilitates fat transport and "serves as the parent compound from which bile is manufactured." And he adds, "The more fat you eat—the more bile you need to solubilize it—the more cholesterol your liver makes" [56, p.239].

Dr. Bortz, though, warns against too much of it and delegates it to our doctor to find out how much is too much. As an insider, he warns us not to become very excited about treatment because "The docs haven't been very effective, and in my opinion, we never will be" [56, p.239]. Especially, if we exercise a lot, the fat will be "burned for energy" [56, p.240], and we will be all right. Thank you, Dr. Bortz, it's good to know.

It seems we are stepping on the path to enlightenment. Dr. C. Norman Shealy, MD, Ph.D., in his book, *Life Beyond 100*, published in 2005, communicates to us his insights on cholesterol. Expanding on the health benefits of the Dehydroepiandrosterone DHEA hormone, he says, "I consider DHEA, the most abundant hormone in the human body, also to be the single most important chemical in evaluating health and longevity. As with most hormones, it is manufactured from cholesterol in the body..." [57, p.33].

He shows that he is familiar with the lipid peroxidation issue, saying, "Most free-radical damage is in the cholesterol/lipid structures of the body. Thus, lipids that have been converted into free radicals are the results of lipid peroxidation" [57, p.52].

As a medical doctor himself, he is not inclined to play cholesterol games, telling us, "There is no circumstance under which I would take any of the cholesterol-lowering drugs. They are dangerous, and it is another experiment like Prempro® that may not be revealed until thousands have suffered complications and/or death" [57, p.181].

Dr. Shealy is a super star in my documentary, *The Secrets of the Longevity Personality,* and told me in a personal communication that he is Blood Type A. I don't know if he is A1 or A2. Most likely, A2 because his parents and grandparents lived to their 90s and 100s, as he said in my interview with him, and himself he is in his early 80s now. In his *The Shealy Commonsense Diet,* he favors meats of all kinds, cheese, eggs, nuts, cereals, legumes [49, p.81-2], butter, olive and coconut oil for cooking, and peanut butter [57, p.174-5]. Except for nuts, cereals, legumes, and peanut butter, his diet is in agreement with my Blood Type A1 diet.

Dr. Joel D. Wallach, DVM, ND and Dr. Ma Lan, MD in their book, *Dead Doctors Don't Lie*, impart to us that, "Elevation of cholesterol above 270 mg per 100 ml of blood is a sign of increasing risk for cardiovascular disease, diabetes, and liver disease (including gall-stones)." Also, "CAUTION: Low cholesterol below 200 can be equally or more dangerous than elevated cholesterol" [58, p.306].

While interviewing him for my film "*Dr. Joel Wallach: From Doctors with Love,*" I asked him about grains, and he replied, "We weren't really big on grains and cereal, never had cereal for breakfast, always eggs and beets, sweet potatoes, as opposed to toast."

Another super star in my film, *The Secrets of the Longevity Personality,* is Brian Clement, NMD, PhD, one of gurus of the vegan raw food movement. In his book, *Longevity: Enjoying Long Life without Limits,* Clement shares with us his wisdom pointing out, "Many of us attempt to avoid the necessary nutrient called fat. This is counterproductive, although it is wise to avoid the saturated fats that are plentiful in dairy products, meat, almost all processed and fried foods and even some margarines" [59, p.34].

Clement considers sprouts of flax, hemp, sunflower, almonds, pumpkin seeds, and chickpeas to be the best sources of essential fats that are necessary for our health. Additional healthy fatty acids for our brain can be obtained from corn, borage, and primrose oil, as well as blue-green algae. He adds, "Such hearty nuts as walnuts, macadamias and pecans contribute significantly to your supply and reserve of essential fatty acids" [59, p.35].

In another of his books, *Supplements Exposed* , Clement warns about health hazards of fish oil, making clear to us that, "The problem is that fish oil is very unstable, and begins to oxidize or decay as soon as it is extracted from the fish and exposed to oxygen, light, or heat. These rancid oils are known carcinogens" [60, p.105]. Clement's message is clear—fats from plants are good, from animal sources, bad. It sounds like, to him, plant-based oils do not oxidize or become rancid. However, the research literature on oil oxidation suggests otherwise.

4

LIPID PEROXIDATION

Fats and oils (or lipids) are subject to oxidation which damages them and decreases their safety, quality, and nutritional value. The degradation products such as peroxides and hydroperoxi-☐ des formed in the process of oxidation not only produce rancid odors and unpleasant flavors, but are potentially toxic and increase health risks including development of various cancers [61]. Lipid oxidation, also known as lipid peroxidation, is defined as, "the destruction of unsaturated fatty acids." Also, "The peroxides set off a chain reaction resulting in membrane, organelle, and cellular destruction" [62, p.51].

The oxidation of PUFAs "...generates hydroperoxides and endo-peroxides that can undergo fragmentation to produce a broad range of reactive carbonyl compounds" [63]. To add insult to injury, as the saying goes, "...the carbonyl compounds can be more destructive than free radicals and may have far-reaching damaging effects both within and outside membranes" [63].

In a Chinese study on the oxidative stability of 18 vegetable oils, researchers looked at their fatty acid composition in relation to Peroxide Value (PV), "a measure of the concentration of peroxides and hydroper-oxides formed in the initial stage of lipid oxidation" [61]. Oils tested in the Chinese study, their ω-3 (n-3), ω-6 (n-6), PUFA, PV values, and the Peroxidabilility Index PI (double-bond index) are shown in Table 15-1.

Table 15-1. Polyunsaturated Acid Composition of 18 Oils

%	Palm	Ca mel lia	Blend 1	Blend 2	Al mond	Zan thoxy lum	Rape seed	Blend 3	Blend 4
n-6	10.1	13.0	15.9	18.9	22.6	15.5	17.5	30.8	35.8
n-3	0.42	1.07	1.07	1.06	0.17	9.55	9.67	1.04	1.03
PUFA	10.5	14.5	17.0	20.0	22.8	25.1	28.3	31.9	37.0
PI	11.0	17.4	19.8	22.9	24.7	37.2	38.2	34.7	39.8
PV	19.5	25.0	25.1	24.5	26.5	26.0	27.5	27.0	27.0

Table 15-1. Continued

%	Blend 5	Pea nut	Blend 6	Se sa me	Corn	Blend 7	Blend 8	Soy bean	Sun flo wer
n-6	37.9	37.9	43.9	45.5	47.5	50.9	54.9	50.8	59.1
n-3	1.03	2.60	1.02	1.58	0.71	1.01	1.01	7.12	0.99
PUFA	39.0	41.2	45.0	47.2	48.5	52.0	56.0	58.1	60.4
PI	41.8	47.1	47.8	50.5	50.0	54.8	58.7	65.8	63.1
PV	27.0	27.5	27.4	27.8	28.5	31.0	32.0	33.0	38.1

Oils are arranged in a way that PUFA values increase from left to right. I calculated Peroxidability Index (PI) using the equation proposed by Arakawa and Sagai [64]:

PI=(% monoenoic FA × 0.025) + (% dienoic FA × 1) + (% trienoic FA × 2) + (% tetraenoic FA × 4) + (% pentaenoic FA ×6) + (% hexaenoic FA × 8),

where monoenoic are fatty acids with one double bond, dienoic-two double bonds, trienoic-three, and so forth. It takes into account the exponential susceptibility of fatty acids to oxidation with each increasing double bond, e. g., oils having two double bonds (n-6) are 40 times more oxidizable than one double-bond oils (monounsaturated MUFAs), three double bonds (n-3)-80 times, and so forth to 320 times for Docosahexaenoic acid (DHA) with its 6 double bonds.

The PI value in Table 15-1 is the lowest of 11.0 for palm oil and the highest of 63.1 for sunflower oil and follows pretty much the pattern of PUFA values, both increasing about 6 times from the lowest to the highest numbers. Camellia and almond oils are closer to the bottom, canola and peanut oils –in the middle, and sesame, corn and soybean oils are closer to the top of the range.

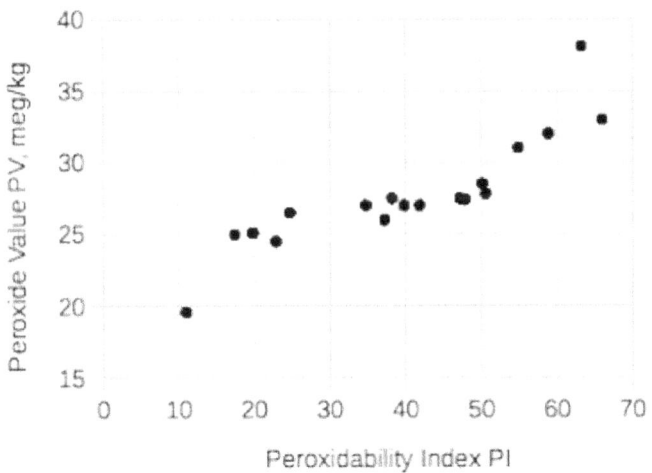

Figure 15-1. Peroxide Value PV vs. Peroxidability Index PI for 18 Oils (Chinese Study).

The peroxide value PV was both measured and calculated in the study [61] and I plotted it on Figure 15-1 as a function of the peroxidability index (PI).

We can see a growth of PV with the increase of PI, which means that the higher the PUFAs (closely match with PI) content of the oil, the more readily it becomes oxidized, rancid and toxic. Peanut oil is in the middle of the PUFA (41.2%) and PI (47.1) range of these values and is definitely subject to oxidation.

Gary Taubes in his book, *Why We Get Fat*, for weight loss advises, "All fats and oils, even butter, are allowed. Olive oil and peanut oil are especially healthy oils and are encouraged in cooking. Avoid margarine and other hydrogenated oils that contain trans fats" [65, p.231]. I wonder if Taubes is familiar with the fat oxidation issues since in the index of his book there is no "lipid peroxidation" or "fat oxidation" entries. Also, among all oils that he allows, some contain *trans* fats produced in the process of their refining and deodorization. Thus, I would take his advice with a grain or two of salt.

A Korean study investigated 10 edible oils and their oxidation products, notably, Malondialdehydes (MDA) [66]. Malondialdehyde is viewed as "an aldehyde formed as a breakdown product of peroxidized polyunsaturated lipids in the body. Malondialdehyde is a mutagen, carcinogen, and cross-linker" [67, p.797].

The vegetable oils tested in the Korean study, their omega-6, omega-3, total PUFA, the Peroxidabilility Index PI, and MDA values are shown in Table 15-2.

The PUFA increases from the lowest 4.94% for olive oil to 61.4-61.5% for perilla oil and both PI and MDA generally follow the trend, although with some exceptions: grape seed oil with its PUFA of 56.2% has 3 times less MDA level (62.8 µg/g) than canola oil (187.5 µg/g) with its PUFA of 20.4%. Also, the MDA values for perilla oil (both industrial and traditional) are disproportionally greate r than for oils close to it in the PUFA content (soybean and grape seed oil).

A marked discrepancy (up to 18 fold) in the omega-3 (n-3) content can be observed between the Chinese and Korean studies for soybean and canola (rapeseed) oils. They are 7.12% and 9.67% in the Chinese and 0.42% and 0.52% in the Korean studies, correspondingly. The United States Department of Agriculture (USDA) value for soybean oil is 6.8% [68] and for canola oil is 9.1% [69], or of the same magnitude as in the Chinese study and 16-18 times greater than the Korean numbers.

Table 15-2. Polyunsaturated Acid Contents of 10 Vegetable Oils

	Olive	Hazel nut	Functio nal	Canola	Sesame Industrial	Sesame Traditional
n-6, %	4.65	10.4	10.5	19.9	34.2	34.6
n-3, %	0.30	0.21	0.37	0.52	0.45	0.43
PUFA, %	4.95	10.6	10.8	20.4	34.6	35.1
PI	7.1	12.8	12.4	22.51	36.1	36.4
MDA, µg/g	50.4	36.5	124.0	187.5	56.4	83.0

Table 15-2. Continued

	Corn	Red Pepper Flavored	Soy bean	Grape seed	Perilla Industrial	Perilla Traditional
n-6, %	44.4	48.3	49.1	56.0	11.4	11.9
n-3, %	0.37	0.43	0.42	0.17	50.0	49.6
PUFA, %	44.8	48.7	49.5	56.2	61.4	61.5
PI	45.9	49.8	50.3	56.95	111.9	111.6
MDA, µg/g	85.5	172.8	180.7	62.8	1080.3	1087.2

Despite the low omega-3 values for these two oils, their MDA level of 180.7-187.5 µg/g is the highest among the other nine oils (except camellia oil), which makes them unsuitable for human consumption. Actually, all oils in both studies are unhealthy and I would use only palm oil. In Figure 15-2, the MDA values are plotted as a function of peroxidability index (PI).

This graph demonstrates that with the increase of PI numbers, the MDA scores also get higher. The researchers of the Korean study observed that "the MDA contents detected in the oils were proportionally correlated to the PI of the oils (r=0.890), *e.g.*, the olive oils and hazelnut oil that presented the lowest PI values produced the lowest amounts of MDA (each 50.4 and 36.5 µg/g), while the perilla oils that presented the highest PI generated the highest amounts of MDA without regard to the oil processing method (1,080.3 µg/g for industrial and 1,087.2 µg/g for traditional)" [66]. They concluded that the PI values "could be used as a predictor for initial oxidation state or quality of the vegetable oils."

Using the USDA database [68, 69], I analyzed the PUFA content of 38 vegetable oils, nuts and seeds, including 5 animal fats (in butter, eggs, lard, beef tallow, and goat cheese), 12 sprouts and greens, 22 grains, and 11 fish oils and seafood items. PI values for oils and fats are shown in Figure 15-3 as a function of PUFA content.

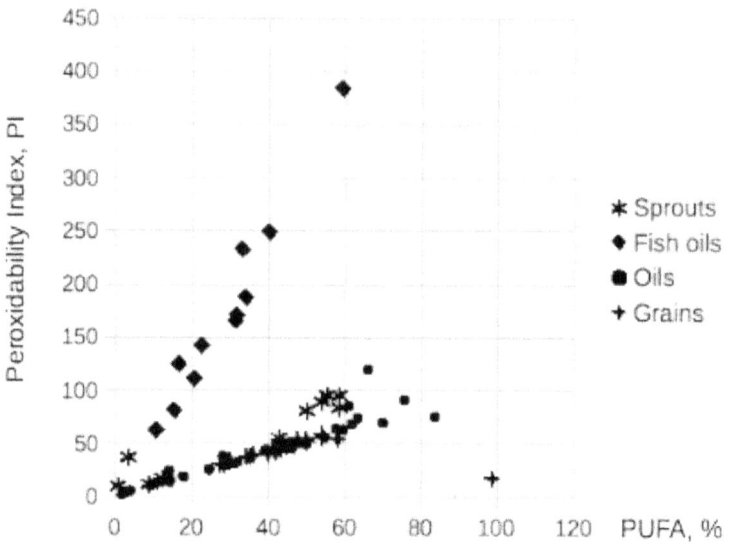

Figure 15-3. PI vs PUFA for 4 Groups of Oils

As we can see, all four groups display an ascent of PI with the increase of PUFA. However, if oils, grains, and sprouts reveal a similar pattern of the PUFA-PI relationship, PI of fish oils soars 5 times faster —PI of 250 versus 50 for 40 % PUFA. The PI values are greater in fish oils because in addition to linoleic acid (omega-6, 2 double bonds) and linolenic acid (omega-3, 3 double bonds), they contain eicosapentaenoic acid EPA (5 double bonds) and docosahexaenioc acid DHA (6 double bonds) which make them exceedingly susceptible to oxidation and rancidity.

Among oils and animal fats, coconut oil had the lowest PUFA content of 1.8%, followed by macadamia nut oil (2.2%), butter (3.7%), and beef tallow (4.0%). These four oils and fats are at the core of my Blood Type A1 diet. On the upper PUFA extreme are evening primrose oil (83.5%), hemp seed oil (75.5%), grape seed oil (69.9%), and flax seed oil (66.0%). Olive oil that is a cornerstone of the Mediterranean diet has 10.5% PUFAs and I do not use it.

I happened to buy a can of the first cold pressed, certified organic extra virgin olive oil, the product of Nu   ñes De Prado company of Spain, and it had a very distinct rancid smell and off-flavor bitter taste. Flax seed oil that is all the rage in the health enthusiasts circles, due to its extreme toxicity, is able to kill cancer cells by means of the lipid peroxidation mechanism [70]. Of all plant-derived oils, **flaxseed oil** has the highest (53.3%) level of α-linolenic (omega-3) acid and its PI value is 119.8 (the uppermost round dot in Figure 15-3).

In the sprouts and greens group in Figure 15-3, parsley has the lowest PUFA level of 0.8% followed by dill (9.1%), and cilantro (12.5 %). Their PI values are 9.5, 11.6 and 17.3, respectively. Navy bean sprouts and alfalfa lead the pack and have the greatest PUFA content of 58.6%, followed by the pinto beans (55.6%). Their respective PI numbers are 95.5, 83.6, and 95.4. Wheat grass (43.1% PUFA, 45.1 PI) and pea sprouts (42.9% PUFA, 55.5 PI) are in the middle of the spectrum.

There are no grounds for Dr. Clement's notion that oils from sprouts are good for us because they also oxidize as any other vegetable oil and become rancid and spoiled even faster considering their exposure to oxygen while growing and in the process of making juices from them or in salads.

In the grain group, white rice has only 0.2 g of total fat in 100 g, of which 28.6% is PUFA, is at the bottom of the whole range and popcorn (58.1% PUFA)-at the top, followed by quinoa-54.1% PUFA. The PI scores are 30.4 for white rice, 54.6 for popcorn, and 59.2 for quinoa. Whole oats have 36.2% PUFA and 39.1 PI. Brown rice contains 1.0 g PUFA in 100 g, or five times more than white rice. Also, it is chewy and I do not use it in my diet.

For many people, the first meal of the day is oat cereal with milk for their breakfast. Dr. Bob Delmonteque, ND, a close friend of Jack LaLanne, was a fitness model and bodybuilder for most of his life until he died at the age of 85. He was regarded as having the best physique in the world even when he was in his 80s. He became very famous for his weight lifting and weight loss promotion career, also he was a personal trainer of Hollywood stars, notably John Wayne, Burt Lancaster, Marilyn Monroe, and American astronauts.

Dr. Bob, as he liked to be called, in his book, *Lifelong Fitness 2004*, advocated eating whole grains, cereals, and starches, less saturated fat, including omega-3s, nuts and seeds. "Polyunsaturated fats are an important part of your diet. Substitute flax seed oil or olive oil for butter,..." [71, p. 165].

Dr. Bob liked my book and we became friends. He learned from our conversations that with my Russian and Japanese background I knew something that he did not know and our phone talks would last for hours. Because I came to this country unbiased and free of the low-fat and "saturated fat is bad" phobia, he was interested in learning from me. For instance, for his breakfast, he had rolled oats, the old Scottish style. When I told him that I opposed eating grains and especially oats, he exclaimed, "How come? Every health expert says oats are good for you." I mentioned that of all grains oats have one of the highest natural fat content. In a study of deposition and subsequent fate of fatty acids in growing oats *(Avena sativa)*, the Swedish and Polish researchers found that "Up to 84% of the lipids were deposited during the first half of seed development, when seeds where still green with a milky endosperm" [72].

Immediately upon their formation, fatty acids became subject to lipid peroxidation in the young grain that was still in the process of maturation. Fats in grains become oxidized, rancid (off-flavor), stale and surely toxic. An even higher PUFA content than in oats is found in quinoa and chia seeds. That is the reason why I do not eat grains, except for white rice which has the lowest PUFA level.

If we take oils in or chew sprouts and swallow them, the oils become further oxidized during the normal metabolic processes inside our body creating additional endogenous toxins [63]. The strategies to minimize the exogenous toxicity of oils like, "Buy oils in smaller rather than larger quantities. Protect them from exposure to air, light, and heat, and use them up quickly" [53, p.149], are of a little help because we have inside ourselves all three oxidizing agents: heat (body temperature of 98.6 degrees F), an oxygen-rich environment, and light. Light in the form of sparkling eyes as raw food enthusiasts gorge on sprouts, and become "enlightened" sucking in their blood (green juice).

Finally, in the fish oil cohort in Figure 15-3, the beluga (whale) has the shortest 10.8% PUFA supply, followed by herring (15.6%), and lobster 16.7%. Their corresponding PI values are 62.9, 81.4, and 124.7. At the richest top is krill oil with 59.5% of PUFA, and not far behind is salmon at 40.3% PUFA, and their PI scores are whopping 383.5 and 249.0, respectively, because of their highest content of EPA and DHA.

Dr. Clement, once lecturing at a health group in Maine, was asked about the claims that some cancer patients benefited from fish oil. He explained that fish oil is protected against oxidation under the water. But as soon as the fish is exposed to the air, its oil immediately begins to oxidize and become toxic. "If you take fish oil, you are insane," was his verdict. He was so right on that. Unlike other longevity gurus, Clement is familiar with lipid peroxidation and its hazards to health, saying, "Lipid peroxide contamination is a condition in which fish oils have oxidized (the oil molecules are destroyed through the exposure to oxygen) and become rancid, cancer-causing fats" [60, p.104].
However, when he recommends oils from sprouts or "...corn, borage, and primrose oil, as well as blue-green algae" [59, p.35], he forgets to mention that they are subject to oxidation too. Corn (54.7% PUFA), borage (61.0% PUFA) and primrose oil (83.5% PUFA) are at the higher extreme of the oxidability range.

As a source of vitamins A and D, cod liver oil that our grand-mothers administered to our parents was believed of doing them good. If grandmas only knew! At this point, it seems relevant to me to refer to a short excerpt from the Russian novel, *Heart of the Dog,* by Michail Bulgakov.

Doctor Preobrazhensky addresses a request to a beautiful girl named Zina, his servant, concerning a street dog that he brought to his apartment,

"Zina! I bought this little scamp some Cracow sausage for 1 rouble 40 kopecks. Please see that he is fed when he gets over his nausea."

There was a crunching noise as glass splinters were swept up and a woman's voice said teasingly:

"Cracower! Goodness, you ought to buy him twenty kopecks-worth of scraps from the butcher. I'd rather eat the Cracower myself!"

"You just try! **If you only knew** what it is made from. That stuff is poison for human stomachs. A grown woman and you're ready to poke anything into your mouth like a child. Don't you dare! I warn you that neither I nor Doctor Bormenthal will lift a finger for you when your stomach finally gives out…"[73].

In the above passage Doctor Preobrazhensky was chastising Zina referring to the poor quality of sausages in the post-revolutionary Russia of 1920s. As far as dogs are concerned, they are carnivores and their biological food is meat. If only grandmas knew what Dr. Ray Peat, a prominent American physiologist, knows about an experiment of feeding cod liver oil to dogs. In his 2006 online article, *Unsaturated Vegetable Oils: Toxic*, Peat shares, "Fifty years ago, it was found that a large amount of cod liver oil in dogs' diet increased their death rate from cancer by 20 times, from the usual 5% to 100%." In the summary of the article, Dr. Peat states, "Unsaturated fats cause aging, clotting, inflammation, cancer, and weight gain. Avoid foods which contain the polyunsaturated oils, such as corn, soy, safflower, flax, cottonseed, canola, peanut, and sesame oil" [74]. These are all oils that the longevity experts mentioned above recommend. **If they only knew.**

5

ANIMAL FAT WILL NOT KILL YOU BUT LOW CHOLESTEROL WILL

There are researchers who knew, something, not all, and were one with Dr. Raymond Peat in implicating PUFA containing vegetable oils with a host of ills such as cancer, atherosclerosis, blood clotting, suppressing of the immune system, cross-linking (loss of elasticity of blood vessels), and initiating free radical chain reactions. They are Durk Pearson and Sandy Shaw, who in their bestselling book, *Life Extension*, published in 1982, unambiguously express themselves saying. "Avoid peroxidized (rancid, autoxidized) fats and oils like the plague!" [67 p.368].

They seem not to fret about cholesterol either when stating, "Substituting polyunsaturated fats for saturated fats, a strategy for lowering serum cholesterol previously recommended by the American Heart Association (AHA) for many years and still recommended by many doctors, is a potentially dangerous practice" [67, p.363]. They sound like describing today's state of affairs, although they voiced it 36 years ago. Conventional wisdom once established becomes regid and slow to change.

In their own diet, Pearson & Shaw favored animal foods, "The two of us together in a week consume: 1 to 2 dozen eggs, about a pound or two of butter, several pounds of beef, poultry, and pork, and 4 to 5 gallons of a whole (not low-fat) milk" [67, p.367-8]. In addition to their hearty diet, they experimented on themselves taking mega-dozes of supplements: vitamins, amino acids, minerals, and food additive antioxidants [67, p.611-3]. They seem to be satisfied with results, "Our own personal experimental life extension formulas have had a dramatic effect on our cholesterol levels. Sandy's total serum cholesterol is 114 milligrams per deciliter and Durk's total serum cholesterol is 91 milligrams per deciliter" [67, p.367].

However, at the time when they were writing their book, around 1980, they could not have known about the later studies in Honolulu published in 2001, the 1997 Leiden, the 2011 Jichi in Japan, and the 2012 Norway studies.

It is amazing how the cholesterol phobia in this country has been so pervasive as to even bring the ancient system of Ayurveda into the fray. Its proponent, Deepak Chopra, MD mentions eighteen studies involving 650,000 people around the world in which "the benefits of having low cholesterol were refuted." He expresses his concern saying, "Yet millions of people have been indoctrinated about cholesterol...," Also, he adds, "The very premise that low cholesterol is beneficial has come under increasing suspicion" [75, p.204-5].

A review published in 1992 included over 100,000 women from a number of countries. "The pooled estimated risk for total cardiovascular death in women showed no trend across TC (total cholesterol) levels" [76]. Moreover, researchers of a Honolulu study of all-cause mortality in 3572 Japanese-American men aged 71-93 years over 20 years found the mortality risk in the group with low cholesterol to be 64% higher than in groups with higher cholesterol [77]. The study also revealed that elevated cholesterol in women was not found to be a risk factor for heart disease.

The Jichi Medical School Cohort study in 12 rural areas of Japan involved 12,334 healthy adults ranging from 40 to 69 years of age. Based on their cholesterol levels, all participants were divided into four groups: <160 mg/dl (low cholesterol), 160-199 mg/dl, 200-239 mg/dl (these two, moderate cholesterol), and ≥240 mg/dl (high cholesterol). After 11.9 years of follow-up, researchers concluded that the low cholesterol group subjects had "hemorrhagic stroke, heart failure (excluding myocardial infarction), and cancer mortality significantly higher than those in the moderate cholesterol group. High cholesterol was not a risk factor for mortalities" [78].

Among Western countries, the Norwegian HUNT 2 study investigated 52,087 participants aged 20-74. Again, all study subjects were divided into four groups according to their cholesterol readings: <194 mg/dl, 195-231 mg/dl, 232-270 mg/dl, and ≥271 mg/dl. The study continued for 10 years and demonstrated that "Among women, cholesterol had an inverse association with all-cause mortality and U-shape" association meaning that the highest mortality rate was observed in the low and high cholesterol extremes. In men also the U-shape association was noted [79].

What was the influence of cholesterol on mortality in advanced age? In a ten-year-long study of 724 people with median age of 89 years at Leiden University, Netherlands, the total cholesterol concentrations were measured and mortality risks accessed. Total cholesterol concentrations were defined in three categories: <193 mg/dl, 194-251 mg/dl, and ≥252 mg/dl. Within the duration of the study, from 1986 to 1996, 642 participants died, mostly of cardiovascular disease, and their mortality risk did not differ among the three total cholesterol categories. However, researchers stressed that "Mortality from cancer and infection was significantly lower among the participants in the highest total cholesterol category than in the other categories, which largely explained the lower all-cause mortality in this category" [80].

Note that the elevated risk of mortality was documented in low cholesterol groups with levels in Japan <160 mg/dl, in Leiden <193 mg/dl, and in Norway <194 mg/dl.

All these studies proved an **increased mortality with the total cholesterol level lower than 160 mg/dl.**

In the Multiple Risk Factor Intervention Trial conducted for "an average of 12 years, 350,977 men aged 35 to 57 years who had been screened for following a single standardized measurement of serum cholesterol level and other coronary heart disease risk factors; 21,499 deaths were identified." Researchers concluded that "For intracranial hemorrhage, cholesterol levels less than 4.14 mmol/L (less than 160 mg/dL) were associated with a twofold increase in risk. A serum cholesterol level less than 4.14 mmol/L (less than 160 mg/dL) was also associated with a significantly increased risk of death from cancer of the liver and pancreas; digestive diseases, particularly hepatic cirrhosis; suicide; and alcohol dependence syndrome" [81].

A study of women aged 50+ years indicated that a cholesterol level of 270 mg/dl was associated with the best longevity [82]. "Mortality was lowest at serum cholesterol 7.0 mmol/l [270.6 mg/dl], 5.2 times higher than the minimum at serum cholesterol 4.0 mmol/l, and only 1.8 times higher when cholesterol concentration was 8.8 mol/l" [82]. This is very important, let me repeat that **mortality** at 4.0 mmol/l (154.6 mg/l) **was 520% higher** than at 7.0 mmol/l (270.6 mg/dl). **Low cholesterol kills.**

Pearson & Shaw's total cholesterol levels of 91mg/dl and 114mg/dl [67, p.367] were very low, and they were aware about possible adverse effects, saying, "It has recently been discovered that some people who have unusually low serum cholesterol levels exhibit a higher incidence of cancer" [67, p.338].

They seemed not to worry about it because, "Our extremely low cholesterol levels are due to high intake of other antioxidants" [67, p.339]. "Other antioxidants" means nutrients or artificial food preservation antioxidants discussed below. To their self-addressed question, "*How long do we expect to live?* " they answer, "...while we expect to live well beyond the normal three score and ten, we can't really predict how long we'll live. Ask us again in 100 years!" [67, p.464].

Three score and ten translates into 70 years [83]. Now, in 2020, they are 77 years old (both born in 1943) and some people are anxious to know how they look. In the video presented on April 29, 2018 they both look fantastic, but when was the video shot, is a question [84].

Discussing oxidation and rancidity of oils and fats, Pearson & Shaw indicate, "In fact, vegetable oils are more dangerous than animal fats because they become hazardously peroxidized (rancid) long before the odor is perceptible" [67, p.378-9]. They see the solution in adding antioxidant food preservatives such as Butylated Hydroxytoluene (BHT), Butylated Hydroxyanisole (BHA), "vitamins E, C, B1, B3, B6, and A, the amino acid cysteine, and the minerals selenium and zinc."

They warn us, "Do not eat any significant quantities of polyunsaturated fats which do not contain antioxidant preservatives such as BHT and BHA" [67, p.371]. It is not clear, however, whether antioxidants will prevent from the formation of endogenous lipid peroxide products from PUFAs as have been discussed previously [63].

It was found in a study of 80 men that supplementing their diets containing "menhaden oil (6.26 g, n-3 fatty acids) or olive oil" (daily for six weeks) with the antioxidant vitamin E (900 IU) did not prevent the release into blood plasma malondialdehyde MDA and lipid peroxide products [85].

Vegetable oils including canola oil are found to be a main culprit of of causing macular degeneration leading to blindness of the 800,000 Australians, according to Dr Paul Beaumont from the macular degeneraation foundation. In people eating vegetable oils, the disease occurs twice as often than in those who don't eat them. As Dr Beaumont said, "Even more convincing was a prospective study where they looked at patients with the disease and those eating too much vegetable oil progressed at 3.8 times the rate of those eating a little vegetable oil" [86].

Although canola oil is touted as "heart-healthy," and advocated by some longevity experts, independent scientists say that "canola oil is a poisonous substance, an industrial oil that does not belong in the body." It contains toxic cyanide-containing glycosides and hemagglutinins. "It causes mad cow disease, blindness, nervous disorders, clumping of blood cells, and depression of the immune system" [87].

Pearson & Shaw demonstrate the effectiveness of antioxidants in extending shelf life of lard, soybean, safflower, and cottonseed oils. They refer to the accelerated aging tests performed by the Active Oxygen Method AOM in which "fat or oil is held at 210 degrees F and exposed to a constant flow of oxygen (in air)" [67, p.378] and the Schaal Oven Test, used in [61], "wherein fats, oils, and food products are subjected to a constant temperature of 145 degrees F (62.8 degrees C) until the first evidence of rancidity can be detected" [67, p.380].

The Peroxide Value (PV), in meg/kg, determined in the AOM test and then is related to the rancid odors "...detected by the nose. This peroxide value is about 20 units for animal fats and about 70 units for vegetable oils" [67, p.378]. It means that the rancid odors in vegetable oils, although present, are much harder to recognize than in animal fats. In the AOM test performed by the marketer of antioxidants, Eastman Chemical Products, the 4 hours for the untreated (control) lard have been extended to 59 hours, or nearly 15-fold, with the addition of Tenox® 0.01% (by lard weight) of mono-Tertiary-Butylhydroquinone (TBHQ) plus 0.01% Tenox® BHA.

In the Schaal Oven test, the untreated lard (control) and safflower, soybean, and cottonseed oils, used for cooking potato chips, revealed delay of rancidity by 6, 4.5, 8, and 10 days, respectively. The greatest delay for rancidity to develop in lard, up to 81 days or over 13-fold, have been obtained with the addition of Tenox® 0.01% TBHQ plus 0.01% Tenox® BHA [67, p.379].

For vegetable oils, the delays were not that dramatic, ranging from 4 days for cottonseed oil (Tenox® 0.02% BHT) to 15.8 days or 3.5 times longer for safflower oil (0.076% Tenox® 6, a mixture of 6 antioxidants and 28% corn oil) to 20 days or 2.5 times for soybean oil (Tenox® 0.02% propyl gallate PG) [67, p.380].

Interestingly, both for lard (11.2% PUFA, 13.3 PI) and safflower oil (14.3% PUFA, 16.2 PI) the postponement of rancidity was markedly greater than for cottonseed oil (51.9% PUFA, 52.7 PI) and soybean oil (57.7% PUFA, 64.6 PI). Much higher levels of PUFA and PI values of the latter two oils render antioxidants less effective. Higher saturated fat in lard (39.2%) and cholesterol could act as an antioxidant.

By its fatty acid composition, lard resembles the fat in human adipose tissue [67, p.379]. Since both pigs and humans are monogastrics (one stomach), and they perfectly transfer fat from the food they eat to their bodily fat and tissues, the composition of their fat is much influenced by the diet [88]. The standard feed of pigs in the mainland America is based on corn and soybeans high in PUFA and its content in the lard of pigs is 32%. In the tropical areas, e.g., Caribbean, pigs are fed with coconuts, low-fat fish and sweet potatoes and their lard contains 3% PUFA or almost 11 times less [27, 89].

In a study of 20 healthy subjects, fatty acid intake was obtained by two 7-day food records and the "influence of fatty acid intake on the fatty acid composition of stored and structural lipids in subcutaneous adipose tissue" was examined. "Subjects with higher intakes of saturated fatty acids exhibited increased levels of total saturated fatty acids and decreased polyunsaturated fatty acids in adipose tissue triglycerides ($p < 0.01$)." Stored triglycerides in human adipose tissue were more affected by diet than the structural lipids, which appeared to be "more resistant to compositional change" [90].

The triglycerides of human adipose tissue are composed on average by 29% saturated, 54% monounsaturated, and 15.5% polyunsaturated fatty acids. "Seven fatty acids predominate as follows (number of carbons: number of double bonds, typical abundance): myristic (14:0, 3%), palmitic (16:0, 19–24%), palmitoleic (16:1, 6–7%), stearic (18:0, 3–6%), oleic (18:1, 45–50%), linoleic (18:2, 13–15%), and linolenic (18:3, 1–2%). These fatty acids account for well over 90% of the fatty acids in human adipose tissue. Odd-carbon fatty acids, longer chain fatty acids, and shorter chain fatty acids account for the remainder. Each of these less-abundant fats individually contributes much less than 1%" [91]. The following will be of special interest to cannibals.

As compared with lard, human fat is 10.2% less saturated, 8.9% more monounsaturated, and 4.3% more polyunsaturated. Both its PUFA content 15.7% and peroxidability index PI of 18.6 are somewhat higher than those of lard, which are 11.2% and 13.3% correspondingly. To decrease both PUFA and PI in human adipose and other tissues an increased intake of **saturated fats** as in coconut oil could be a good idea.

Consequently, it could reduce bringing inside our body advanced glycation end products (AGEs). "High levels of AGEs cause inflammation and oxidative stress, the underlying mechanisms for most chronic diseases, including Alzheimer's disease" [50, p.100]. It can also serve as a strategy for life extension, because, "A low degree of unsaturation (measured as the double bond index and the peroxidability index) of cell membranes is a general characteristic of long-lived species" [63, 92].

Linoleic acid LA (18:2, ω6) is a plentiful fatty acid "in adipose tissue, where its concentration reflects dietary intake." In the United States over the last 50 years, the consumption of polyunsaturated seed oils such as soybean oil high in LA has greatly increased. Based on the review of "studies reporting the concentration of LA in subcutaneous adipose tissue of US cohorts," researchers concluded that, "Our results indicate that adipose tissue LA has increased by 136% over the last half century and that this increase is highly correlated with an increase in dietary LA intake over the same period of time [93].

Linoleic acid in vegetable oils is a substrate (substance acted upon) for lipid peroxidation and free radical formation. In Israel its consumption is "about 8% higher than in the USA, and 10-12% higher than in most European countries."

Together with a high omega-6 PUFA diet in Israel, "there is paradoxically a high prevalence of cardiovascular diseases, hypertension, non-insulin-dependent diabetes mellitus and obesity-all diseases that are associated with hyperinsulinemia (HI) and insulin resistance (IR), and grouped together as the insulin resistance syndrome or syndrome X. There is also an increased cancer incidence and mortality rate, especially in women, compared with western countries" [94].

As was observed in a study in Sweden, the PUFA intake increases the risk of breast cancer. In the course of a 4.2 years-long study of initially cancer-free 61,471 Swedish women 40 to 76 years of age, "674 cases of invasive breast cancer" were documented. Analyzing the influence of different fats in their diet on breast cancer risk, "an inverse association with monounsaturated fat and a positive association with polyunsaturated fat were found." Also, "Saturated fat was not associated with the risk of breast cancer" [95]. The percentage of PUFAs and omega-6 linoleic acid, in particular, were found to be higher in 100 melanoma patients than in 100 matched controls in the 1984-1985 study in Sydney, Australia. "The mean percentage of linoleic acid in the triglycerides of the subcutaneous adipose tissue (PLASAT) of these subjects was substantially higher than that in a similar group examined in 1975-1976" [96].

As noted earlier, dietary vegetable oils are linked to heart disease. In Kerala, India, where coconut oil was a cooking medium, "an average 2.3 out of 1,000 people suffered from coronary heart disease in 1979. During the 1980s due to the campaign against "unhealthy" saturated fat, it was replaced in households by processed vegetable oils. "As a result, by 1993 the heart disease rate had tripled!" [97, p.47]. Are vegetable oils such as canola, corn or soybean oils, really "heart-healthy" as advertised?

6

IS OMEGA-3 HEALTHY?

L ongevity experts and aging researchers contend that omega-3 is a healthy fat based on studies showing that eating fish reduces the risk of heart attacks. They equate fish with omega-3, but it is doubtful that oxidized and rancid omega-3 in fish is a panacea.

Fish, especially warm water fish, are very low in the pro-inflammatory omega-6, 5 mg in cod, 8 mg in tuna, and 19 mg in snapper per 100 grams. That fact or it's low level of the so-called 'problem amino acids' such as *methionine, tryptophan* and *cystine* could be the answer. "While some believe that it's omega-3 fatty acids in fish that protect your heart, others speculate that other fish proteins or micronutrients may be the key" [46, p.200].

Dr. Paster delegates this uncertainty to the 'speculating others,' while himself he is quite certain stating in his book, *The Longevity Code*, published in 2001, "Likewise, consumption of omega-3 fatty acids, found plentifully in fatty fish such as salmon, have a positive effect by reducing the risk of heart disease" [46, p.202].

The same logic is employed by Kris Verburgh, M.D. of the Netherlands in his book by the same title, *The Longevity Code*, first published in 2015 and then translated and published in English in 2018. Referring to the animal and human studies that have showed improvements in such conditions as macular degeneration, rheumatoid arthritis, brain degeneration, Alzheimer's disease, and heart attacks by eating fish or walnuts, he surmises that it was omega-3 contained in these foods that brought about these improvements [98, p.84-85].

Verburgh notes that with the omega-3 supplements such as fish oil, studies show mixed results: some demonstrate a decreased risk of heart attacks, heart rhythm abnormalities, psychoses, and Alzheimer's disease, while other studies show no improvements in heart attacks, Alzheimer's disease or overall mortality.

Verburgh explains the negative outcomes of some studies by the inferior quality of omega-3 supplements that may be "contaminated or oxidized" or other confounding factors such as the use of drugs in trials on heart disease patients. Thus, he advocates omega-3 as a healthy fat and finds support among authorities indicating that "the American Heart Association and the European Cardiology Society recommend a higher intake of omega-3 fatty acids, by eating fish at least twice a week, as well as nuts, flaxseed, olives, avocados, and other healthy food rich in fats." [98, p.86-87].

Dr. Verburgh represents a new generation of the longevity researcher (he was 28 when his book was first published) who does not ride on the 'cholesterol-saturated fat phobia' bandwagon. Talking about Ancel Keys' shoddy Seven Countries Study, e.g. Keys studied 21 countries but picked only 7 that supported his hypothesis, only 9 people were studied in Greece, and eating patterns of only 3.9% of 12,770 participants were analyzed, Verburgh emphasizes that a wrong conclusion had been drawn from this study.

"A re-analysis of the Seven Countries Study done in 1999 shows a more significant relationship between heart attacks and the consumption of sugar, bread, and baked goods, than with eating animal products (which contain saturated fats)" [99]. "How painful is that! Numerous government organizations have based their health recommendations on Keys' views for decades and many still do so today" [98, p.92].

Dr. Verburgh claims to establish a new scientific discipline, nutrigerontology, which aims to retard aging through a healthy diet. He is on the faculty of Singularity University, a Silicon Valley think tank devoted to the development of anti-aging drugs and technologies. Anti-aging methods that Verburgh describes include vaccines and lyso-☐ somal enzymes against protein debris in cells, cross-link breakers, pieces of mitochondrial DNA and CRISPR proteins for DNA repair, stem cells, transfusion of young blood, and epigenetic reprogramming of cells.

All these technologies are currently not in use and it will take years to develop them. "That makes our lifestyle the most powerful instrument we currently have available to slow down aging. Nutrition is the most effective way to slow down the aging process" [98, p.202-3].

Verburgh's diet is based on vegetables, fruits, legumes, mushrooms, nuts, seeds, fish rich in omega-3, poultry in place of red meat, herbs and spices [98, p.209]. Although some animal-based foods are included, in general, they are discouraged and plant-based foods are emphasized. Oats are highly praised and permitted on his diet as well as chia and quinoa.

How important it is to distinguish the workings of omega-3 in **health and disease** is shown in the following examples. Katherine Shanahan, M.D. in her well-researched book (658 references), *Deep Nutrition*, describes her interview with Jo Robinson, a journalist who recalled a "conversation with a friendly Ph.D. candidate" involved in the research on apoptosis (cell death). "Using catheter tubes to directly feed cancerous tumors growing in rats, he discovered that while injecting omega-3 slowed and even reversed the mice's cancer growth, injecting omega-6 accelerated that growth four-fold" [100, p.280].

Dr. Shanahan warns us about toxic, DNA damaging aldehydes such as 4-hydroxy-2-hexanal HHE and malondialdehyde MDA, the products of omega-3 lipid peroxidation [100, p.200]. The focus in her book is on the oxidative damage to omega-6 and omega-3 caused by extrac- tion and heating vegetable oils. She recognizes, though, that MDA can be generated inside our body by its own heat, stating, "It may be the most common endogenously derived oxidation product" [100, p.200].

Nevertheless, she asserts that "...omega-3 helps prevent all manner of disease. Incorporating just a little more of this one essential fat into your diet can help every cell in your body function better" [100, p.281]. It seems that her appreciation of omega-3 comes from the fact that it killed cancer cells in rats/mice.

It did not occur to Dr. Shanahan that omega-3 kills cancer cells due to its extreme intrinsic toxicity and could be beneficial in a **disease** such as cancer, but not in **health** where it can cause "all manner of disease," not prevent them. Ponder this, "A recent trend of balancing high ω-6 intake in the modern diet with increased ω-3 consumption can prove futile if one considers the ω-3 PUFAs as initiators and ω-6 PUFAs as promoters of cancer" [101]. **Omega-3 can initiate cancer.**

Omega-3 was implicated in the development of prostate and breast cancers. In a study of 834 men diagnosed with prostate cancer, researchers found involvement of the long-chain omega-3 and concluded that "This study confirms previous reports of increased prostate cancer risk among men with high blood concentrations of LC ω-3 PUFA." [102].

For the "aggressive" prostate cancer stage, in the Health Professionals Follow-Up Study, increased omega-3 (alpha-linolenic acid) intake was found responsible, "In contrast, for fatal prostate cancer, recent smoking history, taller height, higher BMI, family history, and high intakes of total energy, calcium and alpha-linolenic acid were associated with a statistically significant increased risk" [103].

In the animal model, higher omega-3 intake was found to promote the development of mammary tumors in rats [104]. Feeding rats in their childhood high omega-3 fats (menhaden oil) predisposed them to the development of the breast tumors later in their life. Researchers concluded that "...a high-fat *n*-3 PUFA diet increased mammary tumor incidence; the high-fat *n*-6 PUFA diet had no effect" [105]. Omega-6 in the rats diet was derived from corn oil. For those familiar with alternative cancer therapies, the "Johanna Budwig protocol" of flax seed oil and cottage cheese in the diet had been reported to help many patients [106].

Dr. Shanahan divides fats as good or bad based on whether they "can handle the heat involved in processing and cooking" or not [100, p.132]. Thus, Shanahan likes "...flax, hemp, and other healthy omega-3 rich oils—none of which should ever be used for cooking" [100, p.138]. Even if they are not used for cooking, they are replete with toxic oxidation aldehydes formed in them in the course of their extraction and storage [107]. They are less than healthy, I believe.

You will remember that Dr. Verburgh is not the only one who believes in benefits of omega-3. To base one's trust in something on a few scientific studies, as he and others did, is risky business, though, because science is as a capricious creature as any other woman (in the Russian language 'science' is of feminine gender) and is governed by a woman's logic. That is what science did with omega-3.

On July 18, 2018, the Cochrane Collaboration published the report, *Omega-3 fatty acids for the primary and secondary prevention of cardiovascular disease*, a pooled review of 79 randomized controlled trials RCTs with 112,059 participants. Trials "included adults at varying cardiovascular risk, mainly in high-income countries" and had one to six years duration.

Researchers concluded that "Increasing ALA intake probably makes little or no difference to all-cause mortality (RR 1.01, 95% CI 0.84 to 1.20, 19,327 participants; 459 deaths, 5 RCTs), cardiovascular mortality (RR 0.96, 95% CI 0.74 to 1.25, 18,619 participants; 219 cardiovascular deaths, 4 RCTs), and it may make little or no difference to CHD events (RR 1.00, 95% CI 0.80 to 1.22, 19,061 participants, 397 CHD events, 4 RCTs, low-quality evidence)" [108]. It means that omega-3 (ALA) promoted as a heart-healthy supplement actually makes no difference.

7

SATURATED FAT

The contemporary nutritional paradigm maintains that saturated fat is one of the three villains: the other two are cholesterol and trans fats. "The 2015–2020 Dietary Guidelines for Americans recommends limiting calories from saturated fats to less than 10% of the total calories you eat and drink each day" [109]. The logic of the FDA, American Heart Association, and other nutritional authorities is that "saturated fats raises the level of cholesterol in your blood. High levels of LDL cholesterol in your blood increase your risk of heart disease and stroke" [110].

Walter C. Willett, MD. of the Harvard Medical School, one of the policy makers in the nutrition world, puts it this way, "The traditional link between diet and heart disease is a kind of scientific two-step that goes like this: 1) Too much fat in the diet increases cholesterol levels in the blood; and 2) Higher cholesterol levels increase the chances of having a heart attack or developing some other form of heart disease" [111, p.68]. Willett calls this unproved lipid-heart disease hypothesis [112] "scientific," however, he did not specify what kind of science it is, good, bad or ugly.

We are advised to avoid fats such as butter, lard, and shortening, and "oils that are higher in saturated fat (such as coconut, palm, and palm kernel oils)" [113]. Instead, we are supposed to eat "oils that are higher in monounsaturated and polyunsaturated fats (such as sunflower oil and olive oil) [113] and soybean, corn, and sunflower oil [110]. Also, "The American Heart Association also recommends eating tofu and other forms of soybeans, canola, walnut and flaxseed, and their oils" [110].

Interestingly, canola (Canadian oil) is listed as if it is a kind of seed, bean or nut as its source, from which oil is produced, which is a misnomer. Indeed, canola oil, also known as rapeseed oil, is made from rapeseeds.

Saturated fats, which are abundant in animal fats, dairy products and tropical oils such as coconut and palm oils, are generally regarded as stable with respect to oxidative decomposition resulting in rancidity. Since we are concerned with stability regarding oxidation, oxygen was reported to react with fatty acids at 100 degrees C (212 degrees F) at relative rates: saturated 0.8, monounsaturated 1.1, linoleic 13.7 and linolenic 25.5 (both polyunsaturated fatty acids) [114, p.296].

It means that widely publicized as "heart-healthy," **omega-3 linolenic acid oxidizes 25 times faster** than saturated or monounsaturated fats and easily becomes **stale and rancid.** Rancid oils and fats produce obnoxious and unpleasant odors and flavors, destroy nutrients in foods, and become unacceptable for human consumption. Oxidized fats "promote arterial damage, cancer, inflammation, degenerative disease, and premature aging of cells and tissues" [115, p.89]. Pretty nasty stuff?

As with cholesterol, despite of their unfair bad publicity, saturated fats perform important physiological functions. For instance, **butyric acid** (Butyrate or Butanoic Acid BTA), the short-chain saturated fatty acid with 4 carbon atoms, "...is mostly used as a fuel by the large intestinal cells (often called *colonocytes*) themselves,..." [116, p.46]. Colonic epithelial cells utilize butyric acid as the preferred energy source [117].

Among external sources, rich in butyrate are fermented butter [118] (2.9 g), unsalted or salted butter (2.7 g), cream (1.5 g), and whipping cream (1.2 g), in 100 g of the product [119]. Butyric acid also can be produced endogenously by bacteria such as *Lactobacillus* and *Bifidobacteria* acting on fiber (cellulose) and resistant starches such as green bananas, raw dandelion greens, raw Jerusalem artichokes, which escaped digestion in the small intestine. Both sources considered, "...butyric acid can be derived in large quantities from bacterial fermentation of dietary fiber in the bowel and is also a component of bovine milk" [120].

Studies show that butyrate can protect the colon against cancer development [121]. "Butyric acid can also modify the differentiation state of cells, and in the case of cancerous colonic cells overcomes their resistance to normal programmed death" [120]. In the 2011 study by Tang, Y. et al., the saturated Short-Chain Fatty Acids (SCFAs), including acetate, propionate and butyrate, found to exert their anti-tumor effects via a G-Protein-Coupled Receptor (GPR43), which expression have been detected in the large intestine. "Our results suggest that GPR43 functions as a tumor suppressor by mediating SCFA-induced cell proliferation inhibition and apoptotic cell death in colon cancer" [122].

Butyric acid, also contained in ghee (purified butter), is found to improve digestion, calm digestive tract inflammation, and is particularly beneficial for gastrointestinal disorders such as Crohn's disease and irritable bowel syndrome. Ghee made from unsalted butter is highly praised in Ayurveda for enhancing agni (digestive fire). "It also helps digestion because it stimulates the secretion of digestive juices" [123, p.135]. The aging Blood type A1 people need this digestive aid the most. In addition, "Ghee promotes the healing of wounds and alleviates peptic ulcer and colitis" [123, p.136].

Crohn's disease is a chronic, inflammatory disorder that commonly impacts the lower part of the small intestine and the first part of the large intestine, but can affect the entire digestive tract. It is characterized by painful inflammation of the lining of the GI tract, frequent diarrhea (up to 10 to 29 times a day), rectal bleeding, weight loss, malnutrition, and joint pain.

A 2005 study by Di Sabatino, A. et al. found that oral butyrate "may be effective in inducing clinical improvement/remission in

Crohn's disease" [124]. In a 2013 study by Pituch, A. et al., butyric acid administration was able to reduce inflammation in the gut and soothe pain during bowel movements of the patients [125]. In sufferers of Crohn's disease, "Treatment with butyric acid, a monounsaturated fatty acid, reduces inflammatory conditions, reduces seepage of undigested food particles, and aids in the repair of the mucosal wall" [126, p.219].

In this citation, butyric acid which is a saturated fatty acid is erroneously indicated as a "monounsaturated fatty acid." It reflects deeply engraved fear of saturated fat that the authors (James E. Balch, MD and Phyllis A. Balch, CNC) share with many other nutritional authorities of the day, "The liver uses saturated fats to manufacture cholesterol. Therefore, excessive dietary intake of saturated fats can significantly raise the blood cholesterol level, especially the level of low-density lipoproteins (LDLs), or "bad cholesterol." [126, p.5].

Dr. Peter J. D'Adamo describes a case history of successful treatment with butyrate of Crohn's disease in one of his Blood type O patients, Yehuda, 50 (in 1992), who "already had several bowel surgeries to remove sections that were obstructing his small intestine." Yehuda's condition "...consistently improved. To this day he continues to be asymptomatic" [11, p.276]. "To this day" relates to 1995-6, the time of the D'Adamo book writing, or 3-4 years later.

The laboratory stool butyrate test indicates the presence of friendly bacteria in the intestines capable of prodicing a proper amount of butyric acid. Dr. Jonathan V. Wright, MD reports on a case of Mr. Allenton, 57, with a family history of colon cancer, whose stool test revealed a low butyrate level. Dr. Wright prescribed garlic and goldenseal both of which "inhibit the growth of a variety of unfriendly micro-organisms, and promote the growth of many friendly ones." His patient's second follow-up analysis showed that "... the level of stool butyrate rose to a more normal level, adding another significant factor to his colon cancer prevention program" [32, p.545-9].

A similar increase of the fecal level of Short-Chain Fatty Acids (SCFAs) including butyrate was observed in a four-week study in 16 males and 30 females, aged 31-66 on a diet high in Resistance Starch

(RS) (22 g of RS per day) or Non-Starch Polysaccharides (NSP). Examples of resistant starch include unripe bananas or raw dandelion greens. "Overall, acetate, butyrate, and total SCFA concentrations were higher when participants consumed RS compared with entry and NSP diets, but individual responses varied." Researchers concluded that supplementing the diet with resistant starch "may help maintain colorectal health" [127].

Because of its distinct pungent smell, pure butyric acid is not very palatable. This obstacle can be overcome if butyric acid is administered in a micro-encapsulated form, which also prevents its absorption in the upper part of the gastrointestinal tract and delivers it to the colon where, as in the case of Irritable Bowel Syndrome (IBS), it is needed the most. The common symptoms of IBS are abdominal pain, flatu-lence, bloating, diarrhea alternating with constipation, and mucus in the stools. Women are afflicted twice as often as men. [126, p.354].

In a study of "66 patients with IBS who were given micro-encapsu-lated butyric acid at a dose of 300 milligrams per day...," marked improvements were observed. "After 12 weeks, subjects in the butyrate group experienced decreases in the frequency of spontaneous abdom-inal pain, postprandial abdominal pain, abdominal pain during defeca-tion and urge after defecation" [128]. Definitely, butyric acid helped to improve the quality of the IBS patients' life.

The ability of SCFAs including butyrate along with probiotics to normalize colon environment can be beneficial for obese as well as people with type II diabetes whose gut bacteria is disturbed [129]. On an animal model, "after five weeks of treatment with butyrate, obese mice lost 10.2 percent of their original body weight, and body fat was reduced by 10 percent" [130].

With all these health benefits of butyric acid, does it promote longevity? It seems it does, since its discoverer, Michel-Eugène Chevreul (1786-1889), a French chemist who identified it in 1814, lived to the age of 102 years plus [131]. It is only anecdotal evidence, but it supports the idea of eating butter and ghee regularly. The contents of butyric acid in 100 g of butter (total fat 81.1 %) is 3.2 g [132] and only half an ounce (14 g) of butter a day will provide over

300 mg, the amount that helped patients with IBS in the above mentioned study [128]. Nina Teicholz, an attractive woman and the author of the bestselling book, *The Big Fat Surprise: Why Butter, Meat & Cheese Belong in a Healthy Diet* [133], will approve of your daily butter. Bon Appétit!

The evidence that saturated fat does not cause heart disease is plentiful. Edward R. Pinckney, MD and Cathey Pinckney in their book, *The Cholesterol Controversy* published in 1973, discuss the studies of populations that live on a high saturated fat diet and have low incidences of heart disease.

One of them is the Pennsylvania community of Roseto which was studied for 11 years. "Not only do the people of Roseto eat a great many foods fried in lard (an almost totally saturated fat extremely high in cholesterol), but they also eat their prosciutto ham with a rim of saturated, cholesterol containing, fat more than an inch thick" [134, p.32].

What were their blood cholesterol levels? In men, the range was "from a low of 136 to more than 500, with the average being 224. The women's cholesterol levels were almost identical." Yet Roseto residents experienced less than half deaths from heart attacks than people in nearby cities and in the US as a whole.

Another population was Polynesians in the Cook Islands of the South Pacific subsisting on foods high in saturated fats. One group eating "12 times as much saturated fats as their neighbors show no difference in heart attacks, which are extremely low in both populations" [134, p.33]. Yet another study of the natives in the Punjab region of India reputed to have a diet "extremely high in saturated fat" found that their average blood cholesterol level was 186 [134, p.33].

One more group of people studied for three years were mountain dwellers in Switzerland. "They regularly drink 50 percent more milk, eat four times as much cheese, three times as much lard, use twice as much shortening and about half as much margarine and oil in cooking as do their city counterparts" [134, p.33-4]. The blood cholesterol levels of these rural people was found to be significantly lower than those of city residents.

Russel L. Smith, PhD in his book, *The Cholesterol Conspiracy* published in 1993 analyzes dozens of studies from 1952 to 1985 in which saturated fats were replaced with polyunsaturated fats. He maintains, "In summary, the above studies leave no doubt whatsoever that the consumption of polyunsaturated fats reduces blood cholesterol level" [135, p.194].

Does this do us any good? Not quite, as Smith points out, "Some 31 studies, including Framingham, the Seven Countries study and the large MRFIT study, reported higher cancer or total death rates with individuals having lower blood cholesterol levels." Also, "Eleven studies did not find such a relationship" [135, p.94].

Many studies found that PUFAs consumption is linked to the development of cancer by suppressing our immune system [136]. In addition, high levels of PUFAs "alter the membranes of the body's cells, this also provides a basis for introduction of carcinogens. Still a possible third contributor to cancer is the process of "auto-oxidation" of polyunsaturated fatty acids. This process, involving the combining of oxygen and polyunsaturated fats, results in peroxide free radicals that can cause cells to become cancerous" [135, p.96]. For example, the prevalence (up to 2-3 times) of gastric cancer among males in Iceland, Norway, Sweden, and Japan than that of U.S. males was attributed to their high intake of PUFAs from fish [137]. "Such cancer is probably due to the fact that the toxic peroxides bind strongly to gastric mucosal cells" [135, p.96].

Dr. Malcolm Kendrick in his book, *The Great Cholesterol Con,* published in 2007, looks at "spectacular studies contradicting the idea that saturated fat causes heart disease" [138 p.71]. In a 6.6 year-long study of 28,098 middle-aged men and women in Malmo, Sweden, it was found that, "Saturated fat showed no relationship with cardiovascular disease in men. Among women, cardiovascular mortality showed a downward trend with increasing saturated fat intake, but relative risk reductions did not reach statistical significance" [139].

It means, Kendrick explains, "there was no difference" [138, p.71]. In another randomized, interventional, controlled clinical study (the gold standard) of 48,835 US women aged 50 to 79 that lasted for 8.1

years, two years before the end of the study, the intervention group was consuming 9.5% saturated fat and control group 12.4%. The findings were, "Among the study population as a whole, there were no significant differences in CHD or stroke incidence, CHD or stroke mortality, or total mortality" [138, p.72]. The CHD stands for the Coronary Heart Disease.

Sherry A. Rogers, MD in her book, *The Cholesterol Hoax* announces, "That's why I prefer the whole product, closest to what God created, **Cod Liver Oil**, which contains also vitamins A and D" [140, p.160]. Well, it contains ... But you will recall that dogs receiving cod liver oil all became dead [74].

The "animal fat is bad" consciousness created a number of paradoxes that complicate our less than easy lives even more. To the well known French paradox, a nation with low heart disease despite its high-fat diet, and the Israeli paradox discussed previously, we need to add Italy, Spain, Switzerland, and Japan paradoxes where the increase in consumption of animal foods such as meat, eggs, milk, seafood and saturated fats in recent decades accompanied a "remarkable reduction" in death rates from heart disease and stroke [141, p.79].

Yoshinori Koga of Japan reported that in one farming village fat intake increased from 6% measured 35 years earlier to 22% of calories. "Mean cholesterol levels rose in the community from 150 mg/dl to nearly 190 mg/dl, which is only 6 percent lower than the average American values (202 mg/dl as of 2004)" [141, p.78]. This report and the paradoxes in Europe and Japan definitely fly in the face of the "diet-heart disease" hypothesis.

Definitive evidence to support any hypothesis is deemed to come from randomized, interventional, controlled clinical studies. One of them, the Minnesota Coronary Survey involved 4393 Institutionalized men and 4664 Institutionalized women in six Minnesota state mental hospitals and one nursing home.

In this 4.5-year-long trial, which began in 1968, the diet in the treatment group was 9% saturated fat, 15% polyunsaturated fat and 446 mg dietary cholesterol per day, while in control group the levels were 16%, 5% and 166 mg, correspondingly. The treatment subjects received 7%

less saturated fat, 10% more polyunsaturated fat and 280 mg more of dietary cholesterol.

The subjects consumed these diets for 384 days and it was observed that an initial mean serum cholesterol of 207 mg dropped to 175 mg in the treatment group and to 203 mg in the control group. As researchers concluded, "For the entire study population, no differences between the treatment and control groups were observed for cardiovascular events, cardiovascular deaths, or total mortality [142].

Interestingly, the principle investigator of the trial was Ivan Frantz, Jr., at the University of Minnesota, who worked in the department of Dr. Ancel Keys, an originator of the "diet-heart hypothesis." The study results were not published until sixteen years later, after Frantz retired in 1988, because the trial outcome did not support the "diet-heart hypothesis." Other differences were also uncovered, since 269 patients eating the cholesterol-lowering diet in the treatment group died, and only 206 patients died in the control group [141, p.38].

Even more convincing evidence of the health detriments from replacing saturated fats with vegetable oils emerges from the Sydney Diet Heart Study of "458 men aged 30-59 years with a recent coronary event." The control group (n=237) received dietary saturated fats from animal fats, common margarines, and shortenings. In the intervention group (n=221), saturated fats were replaced "with omega 6 linoleic acid (from safflower oil and safflower oil polyunsaturated margarine)."

At the end of this 7-year-long trial, the intervention group had total cholesterol levels decreased (13.3% vs. 5.5%), but all three causes of mortality looked at were higher in the intervention group than in the control group: from cardiovascular disease, 17.2% vs. 11.0%, from coronary heart disease, 16.3% vs.10.1%, and from all causes 17.6% vs. 11.8% [143].

Yet another piece of convincing evidence is found in a two-year-long "corn oil study" of 80 patients with ischemic heart disease. In this three-way study, a control group (n=26) had animal fats in their diet. Two other groups were restricted as to animal fat, but in its place was supplemented with 80 g/day of either corn oil (n=28) or olive oil (n=26). No significant changes in blood cholesterol were observed in the control and olive oil groups, but dropped about 25 mg/dl in the corn-oil group.

Within two years, 6 patients in the control (animal fat) group, 9 in the olive oil, and 12 in the corn-oil groups either died or had re-infarctions. Investigators concluded that, "The serum-cholesterol levels fell in the corn-oil group, but by the end of two years the proportions of patients remaining alive and free of re-infarction (fatal or non-fatal) were 75%, 57%, and 52% in the three groups respectively" [144]. Note that supplementation of olive oil in place of saturated fats appears not as bad as that of corn oil, but the grim outcomes are close between the two.

The PUFA content of olive oil (10.5%) [145] is five times less than that of corn oil (54.7%) [146] but still those are oxidized PUFAs. While growing and maturing on the olive trees, olives are exposed to all kinds of oxidation agents such as light, oxygen in the air, and warm temperatures of the Mediterranean regions, a perfect storm of sorts.

The process of oil extraction and storage for months, if not years, increases its rancidity even further.

When I lived in Israel in 1991-92, I had a job in Gedera, a town south of Tel Aviv. In my leisure time, I liked to walk in the orange and olive groves nearby. It was spring time, orange trees were blooming and the air was infused with such a heavenly aroma that I could not have enough of it. What added to that delight was the sight of slightly pinkish blooming flowers and orange fruits on some trees remaining from the last harvest.

Once I collected a bag of ripe olives fallen from the trees. I did not eat them; they were bitter and needed to be processed by the olive company to become edible. So, I just had a little "taste" of olives. In the USA, I happened to buy a can of olive oil from Spain, and to me, it had a distinct rancid odor and bitter taste. Olive oil is not a part of my diet, I eat only coconut and macadamia nut oils, butter, and beef suet (tallow), these four containing less than 4% PUFA.

As we see from these studies, vegetable oils such as sunflower and corn oils lower cholesterol levels but shorten our life instead of extending it.

8

STABILITY OF SATURATED FAT

S aturated fats in coconut oil raise LDL cholesterol levels [147], however its effect on LDL sub-fractions is different: it elevates LDL sub-class A, composed of large, fluffy particles, which are not associated with heart disease and lowers small, dense sub-class B LDL that is linked to heart disease [148].

These large LDL and HDL particles are associated with "the cholesteryl ester transfer protein (CETP) gene, which is involved in regulation of lipoprotein and its particle sizes." The increased amounts of large particles were found in the blood of exceptionally long-lived people and their offspring [149]. The CETP gene appears to be inheritable and is protective against an array of old-age diseases. "In fact, Barzilai and other researchers have linked the CETP variant to lower risk of atherosclerosis, heart attacks, hypertension, diabetes, age-related cognitive decline, and Alzheimer's disease" [150, p.133].

In a Brazilian study of the toxicity of various fatty acids on B-lymphocytes and T-lymphocytes, which are the primary cells of the immune system response, it was demonstrated that some fatty acids and particularly PUFAs cause cell death via apoptosis and necrosis more than others.

Apoptosis is "an active process of cellular self-destruction, called programmed cell death," which "affects scattered, single cells" through the shrinking of a cell [62, p.74-5]. Necrosis is a process of cell dissolution, of "cellular self-digestion" in which "cells swell and lyse," as of blood cells and bacteria, or in gangrene [62, p.71,73,75].

The fatty acids with the longest carbon chain and an increased double bond number such as DHA (C22:6), EPA (C20:5), arachidonic (C20:4), and linolenic (C18:3) acids exhibited the greatest toxicity. The toxicity gradually decreased with the carbon chain shortening and was the lowest for butyric and other short-chain saturated fatty acids SCFA [151]. The health advantage of the SCFA strikes again.

The great stability (lowest PUFA and PI values) and the abundance of SCFA bring about the incredible healing and health benefits of coconut oil. The indication of stability is a low level of lipid peroxidation products such as malondialdehyde MDA. Feeding rats a diet containing 16% coconut oil decreased the formation of MDA in their livers by 90% within 1 to 3 days. After feeding them for 10 days a diet containing 16% sunflower seed oil, which is high in PUFA, the MDA values returned to their initial high levels [152]. The most striking is a case of a dramatic improvement in the Alzheimer's patient who was asked to draw a picture of a clock and completely failed. After taking coconut oil, he was able to make a more meaningful drawing [153].

The health benefits of **coconut oil** are well established and range from supporting the thyroid gland, increasing metabolism and enhancing weight loss to fighting viral and bacterial infections to improving arthritis and diabetes conditions to ameliorating heart disease and cancer. Intake of coconut oil markedly improved quality of life of breast cancer patients helping to overcome the side effects of chemotherapy, as a study of 60 Malaysian women aged 36 to 64 years had reported [154].

More and more evidence has been accumulated that saturated fats were falsely accused, and the time has come to exonerate them [133, 141]. Another saturated short-chain fatty acid, **caprylic** acid (C6:0) which is found at 2 % in butter, was reported to provide health benefits. It revealed an ability to ameliorate intestinal inflammation by suppressing the release of a responsible protein, interleukin 8, and may be helpful in treating Crohn's disease. Experiments on animal models also observed its anti-bacterial benefits [155].

Lauric acid, a saturated middle-chain fatty acid (C12:0), which is predominant in coconut oil (44.6 %), is known for its antimicrobial properties [156]. Together with other immune boosting saturated fatty acids, breast milk contains about 6% of lauric acid [157]. It is also "effective as an anticaries, antiplaque and antifungal agent" [158].

Stearic acid (C18:0), a long-chain saturated fatty acid, was shown to have beneficial effects on thrombogenic and atherogenic risk factors. In a study of 13 healthy men, the effects of two experimental diets on the ability of blood platelets to aggregate were tested. With the fat content of approximately 30% of energy in both diets, one provided about 6.6% of energy as stearic acid and another close to 7.8% of energy as palmitic acid. On the stearic acid diet, a significant decrease of "mean platelet volume, coagulation factor FVII activity and plasma lipid concentrations" was observed, while on a palmitic acid diet platelet aggregation has significantly increased. Researchers concluded that, "Results from this study indicate that stearic acid (19 g/day) in the diet has beneficial effects on thrombogenic and atherogenic risk factors in males" [159].

Based on these results, one would surmise that the non-O Blood types (including my A1 Blood type) with their tendency to increased thrombi formation [160, 161] can probably benefit from stearic acid rich foods such as butter (10 %), beef tallow (19 %), and lard (13 %). Or, on the flip side, that Blood type Os who have excessive bleeding issues [162] can benefit from extra palmitic acid in foods.

However, it would be a case of jumping to a conclusion based on questionable evidence because of the serious limitations of the stearic acid study—Blood types of the participants were not taken into account. Blood type Os and non-Os could react differently to stearic and palmitic acids. Furthermore, with too small number of subjects (13) chances of randomness in this study are very high.

Of all saturated fatty acids, **palmitic acid** (C16:0), yet another long-chain fatty acid, is probably the most controversial. It received bad publicity because of its effects on raising serum cholesterol concentrations.

For those rare individuals who have inherited excessively high serum cholesterol (hypercholesterolemia) it could be necessary to pay attention to it. For example, Durk Pearson, his father, and grandfather, who died of a heart attack, all had this condition. Curiously, "At the age of 17, Durk's total serum cholesterol was 185 milligrams per deciliter and his physician told him to either watch his diet carefully or to expect a premature death from cardiovascular disease!" [67, p.367].

It was in 1960 and the cholesterol phobia seemed to be already in full bloom. Durk took his doctor's advice less than seriously and included in his diet tons of meat, butter, eggs and milk rich in cholesterol [67, p.367-8], a diet that would make his doctor cringe. Durk is 76 now and seems going strong but it would be interesting to know how long his physician lived.

The World Health Organization (WHO) in its 2003 technical report, *Diet, Nutrition and the Prevention of Chronic Diseases,* states that "The evidence shows that intake of saturated fatty acids is directly related to cardiovascular risk." Consequently, WHO advises "to restrict the intake of saturated fatty acids to less than 10%, of daily energy intake and less than 7% for high-risk groups" [163, p.91].

Although the report acknowledges that not all saturated fats have a similar effect on raising LDL cholesterol, it indicates that "...intake of foods rich in myristic and palmitic acids should be replaced by fats with a lower content of these particular fatty acids." These two saturated fatty acids (together with *trans* fatty acids) were placed under the "convincing evidence" category of increased risk of developing cardiovascular disease CVD [163, Table 10].

In that table, linoleic acid, fish and fish oils (EPA and DHA) are listed under the same "convincing evidence" section but as imposing a decreased risk of CVD. Under the "probable evidence," α-linolenic acid (omega 3) and oleic acid are in the group of decreased risk, stearic acid-no effect, and dietary cholesterol-increased risk. The Report considers PUFAs (linoleic and α-linolenic acids) as beneficial recommending, "Diets should provide an adequate intake of PUFAs, i.e. in the range 6-10% of daily energy intake" [163, p.91].

Palmitic acid is also implicated with its effect to boost metastasis growth in mice [164]. One may argue that for most people it can not be harmful because it is the most abundant saturated fatty acid in human breast milk. A study of breast milk composition among women in Bolivia, South America and the USA showed palmitic acid concentrations of 25 % and 20 %, respectively [157].

Palmitic and other fatty acids in breast milk are endogenously synthesized, absorbed directly from maternal dietary fats, and mobilized from adipose tissue stores. Humans and animals alike produce different fats, including saturated fats from carbohydrates, proteins, and fats in their diets. Their metabolism creates glucose, amino acids and fatty acids which are further broken down to **acetyl-CoA**, an elementary building block from which fatty acids are synthesized in the liver, and to some extent in adipose tissue, by the process called ***de novo* lipogenesis** (synthesis of lipid or fat) [116, p.77-8].

Human adipose tissue contains 19–24% of palmitic acid [90]. The air sacs (alveoli) of human lungs are covered by fats of which 68 % is palmitic acid [15, p.89]. How did these fats get there without WHO's permission? Well, "The saturated fatty acids can be synthesized within the body" [116, p.21]. All of them, including palmitic acid. Raymond Peat, Ph.D., a prominent American physiologist asserts that palmitic acid can be produced by the body from sugar [166].

The polyunsaturated fatty acids, made by plants (in the case of fish oils, made by algae eaten by fish), are less stable than the saturated fats, and the omega-3 and omega-6 fats derived from them are very susceptible to breaking down into toxins, especially in warm-blooded animals.

Other differences between saturated and polyunsaturated fats are in their effects on surfaces (as surfactants), charges (dielectric effects), acidity, and their solubility in water relative to their solubility in oil. The polyunsaturated fatty acids are many times more water-soluble than saturated fatty acids of the same length. This property probably explains why only palmitic acid functions as a surfactant in the lungs, allowing the air sacs to stay open, while unsaturated fats cause lung edema and respiratory failure.

Even monounsaturated oleic acid (C18:1) "can be synthesized by the body, but the body cannot form n-6 or n-3 fatty acids." They must be obtained from the "diet (in small quantities)" [116, p.21]. How small? According to William Lands, 88, a renowned biochemistry researcher and PUFA expert, "Overall evidence supports advising an estimated average requirement (EAR) for *n*-6 linoleate near 0.1 en%, a recommended dietary allowance (RDA) near 0.5 en% and a tolerable upper intake level (UL) near 2 en%. Similar values for an EAR and RDA are appropriate for *n*-3 linolenate"[167]. It amounts to PUFA's RDA value of 1%. My proposed Blood type A1 diet of daily 2270 kcal, contains about 1g of n-3 and 4.5g of n-6 fatty acids or 0.42% and 1.8%, respectively.

It is within the limits of Lands' RDA recommended value for n-3 (0.5%) and a tolerable upper intake level (UL) for n-6 (2%). And it is 3 to 5 times lower in PUFA than 6-10% of WHO's advised value [163].

For example, rabbits, strictly herbivorous animals, synthesize their fat from grass composed of plant cells enclosed in cellulose (complex carbohydrate). Each of our fifty or more trillion cells has mitochondria known as the "power plants of the cell" and responsible for energy production and the endoplasmic reticulum the major function of which is production and transport of proteins and fats [62, p.2-4].

Palmitic acid has its highest content of 43.5% in palm oil (hence the name), followed by beef tallow (24.9%), lard (23.8%), and butter (21.7%), all now exonerated and brought back into a healthy diet backed by independent research [133].

The history of the palmitic acid's benefits or adverse effects is inconsistent. People who are not worried about cholesterol, sing its praise. "As a stem-fatty acid, palmitic acid is used by our bodies to make other fatty acids and is the major surfactant protecting human lungs: 68 percent of the fat covering our lungs is saturated palmitic acid, found abundantly in palm oil, lard, chicken skin, and butter" [165, p.89].

This sounds good in contrast to indications of its potential to raise

LDL cholesterol [165, p.91], which does not sound so good. Dr. Joseph Mercola indicates that both palmitic and stearic acids lower cholesterol levels [158]. I attribute these inconsistencies to reliance on studies that are replete with limitations mentioned earlier, plus studies on questionable animal models. By the way, what were the Blood types of the mice?

The ability of fish oil peroxidation products, namely thiobarbituric acid TBA, to shrink tumors was demonstrated in the animal model. Human breast carcinoma cells were transplanted to female mice. "At 7-10 days after transplantation, the mice were divided into groups and fed for 6-8 weeks one of the following semi-purified diets containing different amounts and types of fat, i.e. 5% corn oil, 20% corn oil, 20% butter, 19% beef tallow/1% corn oil and 19% fish (Menhaden) oil/1% corn oil."

Researchers observed that after 6-8 weeks of feeding, the decrease of carcinoma volume was the greatest in mice fed the fish oil diet, "intermediate in mice fed the butter or beef tallow diets" and the least in mice fed the 20% corn oil diet. "Supplementation of the fish oil diets with antioxidants (vitamin E+TBHQ) significantly reduced the level of tumor peroxidation products and significantly increased tumor volume (P less than 0.05)" [168].

Menhaden oil is modest in 34.2% of PUFA content and 187.2 PI score, and, nevertheless, manifested the tumor-shrinking qualities. If krill or salmon oil with their much higher PUFA and PI values, had been used in that mice study, the results could have been even more dramatic.

It is evident that many health detriments can arise if we consume bad fats such as *trans* fats, PUFAs (omega-6 and omega-3), and even monounsaturated fats (olive oil). We do not harm our organs and tissues if we eat good saturated fats found in coconut oil, butter, ruminant animal fats, which make us resistant to many degenerative diseases and slow our aging.

9

TRANS FATS

As far as playing with names is concerned, fats are ahead of cholesterol which are called "good" (HDL) and "bad" (LDL); fats are sometimes assigned a third name, "ugly." If you recall, the authors of *The Okinawa Program* use all three names and call monounsaturated and polyunsaturated fats good, saturated, bad and trans fats found in hydrogenated oils, margarine, cookies, pastries, pies, and fried foods, ugly.

Caroline Leaf, Ph.D., in her book, *Think & Eat Yourself Smart* does the same—portraying artificial trans fats as ugly ones and calling them the real public enemy [169, p.171-2]. Another emotionally charged label like "the fat of mass destruction" emphasizes their hazardous effects on health [165, p.87]. Trans fats are found in hydrogenated margarines, shortenings and spreads and in virtually all processed and industrially prepared foods such as cookies, crackers, breads, cereals, pizzas, puff pastries, pies, and chips [170].

In their chemical structure, saturated fats have no double bonds between the carbon atoms, with the full amount of hydrogen atoms attached to them, which makes them stable with respect to oxidation. They are solid at room temperature. Monounsaturated and polyunsaturated fats in vegetable and fish oils are missing hydrogen atoms at the carbon double bond sites where oxygen can attach making them rancid and oxidized. "These bonds are points of instability that are vulnerable to attack by oxygen and that can spring into unnatural positions— creating trans fats—if the oils are heated or otherwise disturbed" [53, p.148].

These oils are liquid at room temperature and some, with many double bonds such as flax, hempseed and fish oils, even in a refrigerator. Oil industries were interested in hardening vegetable oils to widen their use and thus hydrogenation technology had been developed. In the process of industrial hydrogenation, the oils are heated and hydrogen atoms under a high pressure are forced to fill the missing gaps converting them into saturated fats and making vegetable oils harder and less prone to oxidation and thus extending their shelf life.

However, these infused hydrogen atoms are placed in the *trans* geometric configuration of the fat's chemical structure, not in the *cis* configuration as in naturally occurring trans fats (bio-hydrogenation in the rumen) present at low levels in ruminant meat, milk and butter [171]. In addition, the industrial hydrogenation pushes double bonds to migrate from their original position, thus further changing oils chemical structure [172].

The examples of Trans Fatty Acids (TFA) from ruminant fats are palmitelaidic acid (C16:1 Δ9t) [173] and vaccenic acid (C18:1 Δ11t) [174]. The major TFA formed by partial hydrogenation of vegetable oils is elaidic acid (C18:1 Δ9t), derived from oleic acid (C18:1). Altogether, 14 trans fatty acids have been identified [175, p.54].

The trans elaidic acid was found in the 198 breast milk samples of Canadian mothers ranging from as low as 0.1% to as high as15.4% (mean value 5.9%) of total fatty acids [176].

It leads to endothelial sloughing and subsequent sub-endothelial exposure that attracts platelets to fill endothelial gaps. Two antagonistic prostaglandin derivatives synthesized by endothelial cells, prostacyclin and thromboxane are involved in platelet adhesion: thromboxane promoting and prostacyclin inhibiting it [62, p.831]. This further leads to the major cause of heart disease, which is oxidized cholesterol and trans fats promote this cholesterol oxidation.

The change in fat's chemical structure makes artificial *trans* fats a challenge to our living cells in terms of their assimilation and utilization. Not only that, they become pro-inflammatory in our body [176] and atherogenic, e.g., promoting the development of atherosclerosis and greatly increasing the risk of cardiovascular diseases [177].

The pioneering researcher who investigated *trans* fats was Fred A. Kummerow, Ph.D. (1914-2017) [178], who first published his article in 1957 in *Science* demonstrating the tissues of heart disease patients having significant amounts of trans fatty acids [179].

According to Kummerow, it is not elevated LDL cholesterol that causes atherosclerosis and cardiovascular disease, but its oxidized form, oxysterol created by intake of trans fat containing fried foods [175, p.34]. The title of his book, "Cholesterol Won't Kill You But Trans Fat Could: Separating Scientific Fact from Nutritional Fiction" [180], reflects his insights.

Kummerow was living proof of the rightness of his health-promoting ideas because he lived to the age of 102, a long and an extraordinarily productive life. I believe his research and unbending will and boldness (he filed a petition to FDA at the age of 98) have saved many lives.

When he turned 101, I sent him an email:

Dear Dr. Fred Kummerow,

Will you still accept congratulations on the occasion of your 101th birthday?

Happy Birthday to You and Many Happy Returns!

You are my hero. I am your fan and follower. I am a Russian born, retired engineer, residing for the last 18 years in the USA. It has always been second nature to me to be passionate about health, fitness, and longevity. Being trained as a researcher, I applied my skills to longevity research, which I conducted in many countries.

It culminated in my book "Control for Life Extension. A Personalized Holistic Approach," and five documentaries on health and longevity, including "The Secrets of the Longevity Personality." www.longevitywatch.com/index.html. In YouTube under my name, my 16 films can be viewed.

My particular interest is food oils, specifically oxidized PUFAs. Avoiding them is crucial for my survival because my Blood Type is A, which has an average life span of 62 years. I am 74 and was able to survive 12 years beyond my average life span because I watch my diet very closely—I do not eat grain products, which I believe are detrimental to the human race (I have proof). My only oils and fat are coconut oil, butter, beef tallow and macadamia nut oil. My diet is nutritionally balanced, I eat meat, eggs, seafood and my philosophy fits into the Yogi doctrine.

I would love to interview you and make a documentary on you.

Thank you very much,

Sincerely, Valery Mamonov.

On her father's behalf, Kay, his daughter, replied:

Thank you for your kind offer of a documentary on my work, however, I must respectfully decline. I am still working full-time at age 101. I already have enough publicity.

Kay (daughter replying for Dr. Fred Kummerow).

DR. MARY ENIG of the University of Maryland joined forces with Kummerow and published articles warning authorities and the public about the detriments of *trans* fats. The Chicago Health and Aging Project, a dementia and cognitive decline study conducted in 1993-2000, demonstrated that an intake of two or more grams *trans* fats a day increased the risk of developing Alzheimer's disease three to five times. Two large factory-made chocolate chip cookies contain that amount of *trans* fats [50, p.95]. This study also found that eating 25 g of saturated fat per day over a four-year period increased participants risk of developing Alzheimer's disease 2-3 times [181].

This trial was an epidemiological (observational) study, lead by Morris M. C., a doctor of epidemiology from the Harvard T. H. Chan School of Public Health. The problem with those kinds of studies is that researchers look for an association between an illness, e.g. Alzheimer's disease and dietary factors, e.g. saturated fat or trans fats, but not causation [133, p.42].

Animal fat as lard or hydrogenated margarines made from vegetable oils could contain both saturated fat and trans fats mixed together, but they do not distinguish between the two in the studies [141]. In the Chicago Project, however, they looked at both trans fats and saturated fat, but, taking into account that Dr. Morris is "anti-saturated fat" by training, how do we know what really caused Alzheimer's disease in the participants diet, trans fat or saturated fat.

Dr. Morris developed the MIND diet for healthy brain aging and tested it in the Memory and Aging Project (MAP), an almost 5-year-long study among 923 Chicago participants aged 58 to 98 unaffected by dementia. She found that her diet is superior to the Mediterranean and Dietary Approaches to Stop Hypertension (DASH) diets in terms of cognitive decline and Alzheimer's disease [50, p. 114].

The MIND diet mimics the Mediterranean diet with a heavy emphasis of olive oil, whole grains (3 servings a day), beans and legumes (4+ servings a week), a glass of wine and a restriction of red meat (<4 servings a week), whole-fat cheese (<1 serving a week), butter or trans-fat margarine (<1 serving per day), and fried foods (<1 serving a week) [50, p.112-3].

Note that butter (saturated fat) and *trans* fats are lumped together as in many politically-correct dietary advice. This diet will be tested in an additional MIND trial ending in 2021 and "will form public health policy and dietary recommendations for healthy cognitive aging" [50, p.115]. She dooms us to age "cognitively healthy" eating grains, legumes and skipping meat and butter.

Defending her "whole grain" standpoint, Morris mentions Dr. David Perlmutter's book, *Grain Brain*, which connects grain consumption with the inflammation prevalent in Alzheimer's disease. However, she discards "Dr. Perlmutter's hypothesis" on the grounds of "scientific evidence" that she gathered from the PREDIMED trial, a parallel-group, randomized study of 7,447 people in Spain.

This trial showed the benefits on cardiovascular events of eating the Mediterranean diet (two intervention groups supplemented with either olive oil or nuts) over a control group with reduced fat, which actually was a low-fat diet [182]. The PREDIMED trial had nothing to do with grains, the intake of which was equal in all three groups, it studied the effects of fats. If Morris herself eats the whole grains that she advocates, they probably badly affected her reasoning, as this example shows and the *Grain Brain* implies.

In the complicated field of nutritional science, one can prove or disprove anything that fits their agenda. As Ancel Keys demonstrated, no matter how biased and unproven their theories are, if they push hard enough, one can climb the mountain of nutritional Olympus and from that lofty perch they can shape public health policy.

What the Olympus policy makers and their opponents agree upon, though, is the health hazards of ***trans* fats.**

The two massive prospective observational studies were the Nurses' Health Study (NHS) of 83,349 "registered female nurses aged 30 to 55 years in 1976" and the Health Professionals Follow-up Study (HPFS) (dentists, veterinarians, pharmacists, optometrists, osteopathic physicians, and podiatrists [111 p.32]) of 42,884 "male health professionals aged 40 to 75 years in 1986" [183]. "Another 116,000 young nurses were enrolled in the study in 1989" [111, p.32]. NHS and its follow up continued from 1980 to June 2012, for 31.5 years and HPFS from 1986 to December 2012, for 26 years.

The studies outcome was that isocaloric substitution for carbohydrates in the diet with 2%   *trans* fats, resulted in an increase of mortality from all causes by 13%, cardiovascular disease by 27%, neurodegenerative disease by 51%, and respiratory disease by 40%. The only disease that mortality was a little lower (by 7%) was cancer [138]. A possible explanation of this discrepancy is that toxic trans fats kill cancer cells in the same manner as chemotherapy or omega-3 in flaxseed and fish oils do.

For each variable analyzed, all participants were grouped into five quintiles. An interpretation of the studies results involved the multivariable-adjusted model that researchers developed. It adjusted for age, Caucasian or not, marital status, body-mass index, physical activity, smoking status, alcohol consumption, for the use multivitamins, vitamin E supplements, current aspirin, family history of myocardial infarction, diabetes, cancer, a subject's history of hypertension, hypercholesterolemia, intakes of total energy, dietary cholesterol and percentage of energy intake from dietary protein, and menopausal status and hormone use in women.

It looks like many confounding factors were taken into consideration to exclude their influence on the determinants under scrutiny, e.g. saturated fat, trans fat, MUFA, PUFA, and carbohydrates. Unfortunately, researchers failed to include other confounders, the most important of which is **Blood type**.

If we assume that both NHS women and HPFS men share the proportions of Blood types with the whole US population [184], than 52.4% (44% O plus 8.4% A2) have a life span of 87 years, 10% (B)–80 years, 4% (AB)– 69 years, and the remaining 33.6% (A1)–62 years [185, p.76].

At the start of NHS study in 1980, women were 4 years older than in 1976, aged 34 to 59 years. Within 31.5 years of the study and follow up, of 83,349 participants 20,314 nurses died, or 24.4 %, nearly a quarter of them. At what age did they die? Did nurses with Blood type A1 die out first? Did they die following the pattern of the Blood type-determined age at death? What are the age and Blood type of the participants that are still alive?

At the inception of the HPFS study in 1986, men aged 40 to 75 years were older than women by 4 to 16 years. By the end of the study in 2012, 12,990 men died, 30.3 % of them. Their death rate was about 6% higher than for women. At the beginning of the study in 1986, among those in their late 60s and 70s (the upper quintile by age), how many were close to or exceeded their Blood type specific life span? In the course of the studies, as participants aged, how many died according to their Blood type life span?

Blood type Os having the strongest immune and digestive systems and thin blood would better resist the staphylococcus infections prevalent in the hospitals [186] than non-Os. As studies continued for 26-31.5 years and subjects developed any type of disease, what kind of treatments did they receive? Within the years of the studies, those participating from the outset were influenced by the predominating dietary advice of their time which was the shift from animal foods and fats to plant-based food, cereals, breads, cookies, margarines, short-ening and refined vegetable oils replete with trans fats–all foods promoting diabetes. Because of this shift to higher carbohydrate intake, how many became overweight and obese?

Diabetic patients were excluded from the studies at their inception, but how many developed it on the way and were prescribed statin drugs which undermined their immune systems? [187]. How many nurses or health professionals were on street drugs? I will not over-whelm you with more questions, if one is inclined, they can continue according to their experience and concerns. In short, if all these factors were taken into account, the results of these studies could be very different.

To add insult to injury, the interpretations of the results of these poorly designed studies are no better. Instead of presenting the number of deaths in each quintile and a suspect factor, e.g. saturated fat or *trans* fat consumed in that quintile, the authors of the study employed the substitution technique: the number of deaths and hazards ratios are calculated if saturated fat, as a major foe, is replaced by the isocaloric carbohydrates or other fats. However, carbohydrates whether whole grains or refined grains with added sugar, which differently impact heart disease [188], are not specified.

This vagueness and statistical manipulation is even hard to grasp for Alice H. Lichtenstein, a Professor of Nutrition at Tufts University in Boston, the co-author of the AHA report, "Therefore, it is critical to the interpretation of findings in nutritional epidemiological studies that the contrast in dietary patterns between high and low saturated fat intake be well characterized. Simply comparing disease rates between people in a population who have low compared with the high intake of saturated fat is fraught with potential for misinterpretation and misun-derstanding" [189].

If Alice does not understand this chicanery, how can we, "just the ordinary people" who "don't know where to go," as the song goes, understand? Because all human observational and intervention clinical studies linking diet and disease, e. g. NHS, HPFS, PREDIMED, DART, Lyon Diet Heart Study, etc., which do not include **Blood type**, are marked by the same cardinal defect. They must be excluded from serious analysis.

Because millions and millions of dollars are spent on NHS and HPFS studies, we will try to glean something from them. The paper on these studies [183] is confined to the analysis of fats and deaths, so the following analysis is my own. Comparison of mortalities in two studies from different causes is shown in Table 15-3.

Table 15-3. Mortalities from Different Causes in NHS and HPFS Studies

Study	CVD		Cancer		NDD	
	Deaths	%	Deaths	%	Deaths	%
NHS	4000	19.7	7919	39.0	2079	10.2
HPFS	3878	29.8	4192	32.3	840	6.5

Table 15-3. Continued

Study	RD		Other	
	Deaths	%	Deaths	%
NHS	1584	7.8	4732	23.3
HPFS	988	7.6	3092	23.8

Legend: CVD – cardiovascular disease; NDD – neurodegenerative disease; RD – respiratory disease.

AS WE CAN SEE from this Table, the most prevalent mortality was from cancer (39 % for women and 32.3 % for men), followed by cardiovascular disease CDV (19.7% for women and 29.8% for men). As opposed to women, many more men died of CVD, but 6.7 % more women died of cancer. How many of them received standard cancer treatments of chemotherapy, surgery, and radiation? How many subjects in both studies that developed cancer and had undergone conventional treatments survived and for how long? In 1980 a total of 88,795 women were cancer-free, but within 4 years of follow-up, 468 (0.7%) women were diagnosed with having breast cancer. The number of cancers increased to 1499 (1.7%) in 1988, and further to 2,956 (3.4%) in 1994, including 784 premenopausal and 1,913 post-menopausal cases. At that time, after 14 years of follow-up, researchers concluded, "In contrast to the predominant hypotheses, we saw no increased risk of breast cancer with increased intake of animal fat, polyunsaturated fat, saturated fat, or trans unsaturated fat in models in which fat intake replaced carbohydrate intake" [190].

Walter C. Willett, M.D., a leading investigator of NHS and HPFS studies, in his book, *Eat, Drink and Be Healthy,* published in 2001, indicates that "In the Nurses' Health Study, more than five thousand participants have developed breast cancer since 1980. So far we have not seen an increase in breast cancer with higher dietary fat. In fact, the rate of breast cancer among women who ate the most dietary fat was slightly *lower* than the rate among women who ate the least" [111, p.91].

How nice! Even trans fats are found harmless. Women were contin-uously developing breast cancer and your fat-carbohydrate-replace-ment model did not find why. How long are you going to puzzle Alice with your model? Did you look beyond fat, at the other possible culpable agents such as mammograms, annual flu vaccines, staph infections in the hospitals that poor nurses are exposed to day-in and day-out? What was women's Blood type?

One would think that these colossal studies cost American taxpayers tens if not hundreds of millions of dollars. Well, much more than that. "The Women's Health Initiative, which is primarily testing the impact of reducing dietary fat to 20 percent of calories and increasing fruits and vegetables on the development of breast cancer, will cost more than $1 billion and still probably won't yield clear answers on this important question" [111, p.30]. Surely, we cannot expect to have clear answers from that sort of funds-hungry shoddy research. The only people who can benefit from these studies are researchers themselves. America is a very rich country, perhaps it can afford such waste.

Nurses who were never diagnosed with heart disease at the beginning of the NHS study in 1980, for the next 14 years, to 1994, had 965 heart events, of which "684 of these women survived heart attacks, and 281 died from heart disease" [111 p.78-9]. Here we go! What if those who survived were Blood type Os and Bs (71%) and who died—type A1s and ABs (29%)? The percent numbers roughly match the US blood distribution, 64%, and 36%, respectively. Because it is hard to kill Blood type Os and Bs and easy A1s and ABs. That fact could be more evident than that they ate more unsaturated fats and less saturated ones, as researchers claim [111, p.79].

Among those who survived and who died from CVD, how many have undergone heart bypass surgery or stents and what was their survival rate? In the "Other deaths" cohort, how many developed diabetes and had their limbs amputated? How many were on kidney dialysis? After they developed the disease, how much had their diet changed? If they were hospitalized, how long did they stay there before death? In the study population, what was an average life span for men and women? We want to know the answers to all these questions.

Over time, the overwhelmingly convincing evidence of profound adverse effect of *trans* fats, based on Kummerow, Enig and others' research, accumulated to the extent that government agencies, despite the resistance of processed food manufacturers, began to take action.

The World Health Organization (WHO) in its technical report recommended trans fats intake of less than 1% of daily energy [163], or less than 2.2 g a day in a 2000 kcal diet. Denmark banned trans fats in 2003 [191]. The U.S. Food and Drug Administration (FDA) issued a labeling requirement for trans fats in 2003, effective January 1, 2006. The packaged food products on their nutrition label must indicate trans fats, if their content is equal or greater than 0.5 g per serving. The food producers were allowed to report zero if trans fats were less than 0.5 g per serving [192]. In the US, the first metropolis to outlaw trans fats was New York city where since 2005 the use of partially hydrogenated oils was not allowed in restaurants [193]. In 2013, Kummerow filed a petition to FDA stating that "Artificial trans fat is a poisonous and deleterious substance..." and urged the FDA to ban it [194].

They seem to take notice and the FDA banned trans fats in the United States on June 16, 2015 [195], giving food producers a deadline of three years. The FDA stressed that trans fat had no GRAS (generally recognized as safe) status and "could no longer be added to food after June 18, 2018, unless a manufacturer could present convincing scientific evidence that a particular use was safe" [196]. Canada followed and announced that trans fat will be prohibited effective on September 15, 2018 [197].

Table 15-4. Fatty Acids and Trans Fats in Corn, Soybean and Canola Oils

Oils, 100 g	SFA, g	MUFA, g	PUFA, g			Trans fats		
			Total, g	Omega 6, g	Omega 3, g	Total, g	Mono enoic, g	Poly enoic, g
Partially Hydrogenated Oils								
1	10.1	71.1	14.0	12.54	1.50	27.0	22.8	4.2
2	14.2	30.3	24.2	21.53	2.64	15.0	14.3	0.7
3	15.2	38.9	24.3	22.34	1.96	14.9	14.2	0.7
4	13.6	33.5	20.2	18.17	2.08	14.8	14.0	0.8
5	11.6	45.3	23.1	15.16	6.18	0.3	0.1	0.2
Deodorized Oils								
6	7.8	61.2	26.4	18.76	9.14	1.8	0.3	1.5
7	7.6	61.2	25.6	17.92	6.40	1.6	0.1	1.5
8	6.5	72.0	17.1	14.50	2.60	0.8	0.1	0.7
9	7.4	63.3	28.1	18.64	9.14	0.4	0.0	0.4
10	8.0	58.5	29.1	22.98	5.80	0.3	0.0	0.3

ASIDE FROM HYDROGENATION, trans fats are also created in the process of deodorization, refining, and deep frying in vegetable oils which is carried out at high temperatures ranging from 180°C to 270°C [198] Table 15-4 demonstrates the presence of trans fats in a few brands of corn, soybean and canola oil formed by both partial hydrogenation and deodorization.

Source: USDA Data Base

1. Oil, vegetable, industrial, canola (partially hydrogenated) oil for deep fat frying [199]

2. Margarine-butter blend, soybean oil and butter [200]

3. Margarine, 80% fat, stick, includes regular and hydrogenated corn and soybean oils [201]

4. Margarine, margarine-type vegetable oil spread, 70% fat, soybean and partially hydrogenated soybean, stick [202]

5. Margarine, 80% fat, tub, CANOLA HARVEST Soft Spread (canola, palm and palm kernel oils) [203]

6. Oil, vegetable, industrial, canola for salads, woks and light frying [204]

7. Oil, industrial, canola with an antifoaming agent, principal uses salads, woks and light frying [205]

8. Oil, vegetable, Natreon canola, high stability, non trans, high oleic (70%) [trans free high stability low saturated fat non-hydrogenated canola oil] [206]

9. Oil, vegetable, canola [low erucic acid rapeseed oil] [207]

10. Oil, corn and canola [208]

As we can see, the highest content of 27% *trans* fat is found in the industrial partially hydrogenated canola oil (1) for deep frying. The fats in margarine made from hydrogenated corn and soybean oils (2-4) incorporate 14.8-15.0% *trans* fat. Among the deodorized oils, canola oil (6-10) contains 0.3% to 1.8% trans fat. In a study of unhydrogenated vegetable oils, it was found that canola oil contains from 0.56 % to 4.2 % *trans* fat [209].

The effects of *trans* α-linolenic acid derived from deodorized rapeseed (canola) oil (57%) and margarine (43%) on blood cholesterol were investigated in the *Trans*LinE Study, a controlled, parallel intervention trial on 88 subjects aged 18 to 55 years from France, Scotland, UK, and the Netherlands. In the treatment group of 44 subjects, in whom the diet was supplemented with 1.41g of *trans* α-linolenic acid for six weeks, the plasma *trans* α-linolenic acid in cholesteryl esters (cholesterol attached to a fatty acid [87, p.14]) increased from 0.11 to 0.36 g/100 g fatty acid, or more than 3 times, but did not change in the control group receiving no *trans* fats [210]. It means that deodorized oils infuse the blood with *trans* fats, which can adversely affect blood vessels.

One can ask, what is a safe amount of *trans* fats in the diet? Consumer advocates have a clear answer, it is **zero** [211]. Consumer, beware! Because *trans* fats are so pervasive, the best strategy is to cover one's head with a blanket and never go out, otherwise, they will get you. "Duck and Cover," as the drills during cold war era instructed. Not to be affected financially, one can demand their employer to pay them the way they do for sick days, as in the case of flu or natural disasters such as hurricanes, tornados, earthquakes, tsunamis, etc. While under the blanket, often repeat after Dr. Richard Schulze, "It's great to be alive!"

10

FATS IN HEALTH AND DISEASE

ealth and disease are different states of an organism and we feel good when we are healthy and not well when we are sick. Illnesses alter physiological parameters and medical tests show deviations from normal conditions. To confront illness, from the beginning of human societies both folk and conventional medicines were created to help our internal environment to return to normal. Nutrition and diet have been long recognized as powerful medicine down to the present day, for example, the Nutrition Medical Therapy [212, p.243] in the treatment of diabetes. Quite a few medical doctors place nutrition at the focus of their treatment with success [2, 352 43, 115, 213]. A clear understanding that nutrition must be different in health and disease will help overcome confusion coming from many food health claims and studies which often have opposite results.

Fat, carbohydrates and protein are three macronutrients constituting our food. Because some fats were implicated in causing heart disease, stroke and cancer, they became the most feared food constituent, espe-cially saturated fat. As we have seen in a previous section, a few saturated fatty acids were proven to have healing properties. Saturated fat's bad reputation is based on the studies showing that they elevate LDL blood cholesterol, however, it was demonstrated time and again that LDL is a poor indicator of coronary artery disease.

Julius Torelli, MD in his book, *Beyond Cholesterol,* describes seven laboratory tests that are much more definitive indicators of CAD than cholesterol: 1. C-reactive protein, 2. Fibrinogen, 3. Homocysteine, 4. Fasting insulin, 5. Ferritin, 6. Lipoprotein (a), and 7. Scan of heart calcium [214]. Note that none of them is the cholesterol test, although elevated HDL cholesterol is associated with a decreased risk of CAD [185, p.19]. Also, elevated LDL cholesterol was found not to increase, but decrease mortality from all causes [77, 78].

Of all fats and oils, the highest saturated fat (92.4%) and the lowest PUFA (1.8%) content is found in coconut oil. The remaining 5.8% is monounsaturated oleic acid (C18:1) [215]. Coconut oil contains a full spectrum of seven saturated fatty acids ranging in carbon chain length from C6:0 (caproic acid, 6%) to C18:0 (stearic acid, 2.8%), with the most abundant lauric acid (C12:0, 44.6%).

Lauric and myristic (C14:0, 16.8%) acids are called Medium-Chain fatty acids or Triglycerides (MCT) and comprise 61.4% of saturates in coconut oil. Other short-chain fatty acids are caprylic (C8:0, 7.5%) and capric (C10:0, 6%) acids. All of its tiny 1.8% PUFA content comes from omega-6 linoleic acid (C18:2) and it has **0% of omega-3 α-linolenic acid** (C18:3). The absence of the latter acid with three double bonds makes coconut oil the **most stable** (Peroxidability Index PI 1.9) fat of all natural oils and fats. Depending on whether fats and oils are solid or liquid at room temperature, they are divided into two groups: solid fats and oils [216]. Examples of solid fats and oils and percentages of their individual fatty acids are shown in Table 15-5.

Source: U.S. Department of Agriculture, Agricultural Research Service, Nutrition Data Laboratory. USDA National Nutrient Database for Standard Reference. Release 27, 2015 [215]. Data in Table 15-5 for individual fats and oils are all acquired from the USDA Database except for krill oil which is obtained from a research paper [186]. Sources [174] through [186] are indicated in references 217-229.

Table 15-5. Content (%) of Fatty Acids in Fats and Oils

Chain Length: Double Bonds	Fatty Acid	Coconut oil	Palm Kernel oil	Butter	Beef Tallow	Palm oil	Lard	Chicken Fat
C4:0	Butyric	0	0	2.6	0	0	0	0
C6:0	Caproic	0.6	0.2	1.63	0	0	0	0
C8:0	Caprylic	7.5	3.3	0.96	0	0	0	0
C10:0	Capric	6.9	3.7	2.05	0	0	0.1	0
C12:0	Lauric	44.6	47.0	2.1	0.9	0.1	0.2	0.1
C14:0	Myristic	16.8	16.4	6.02	3.7	1.0	1.3	0.9
C16:0	Palmitic	8.2	8.1	17.6	24.9	43.5	23.8	21.6
C17:0	Margaric	0	0	0.45	0	0	0	0
C18:0	Stearic	2.8	2.8	0.45	19.0	4.3	13.5	6.0
C20:0	Arachidic	0	0	0.11	0	0	0	0
C22:0	Behenic	0	0	0	0	0	0	0
C16:1	Palmitoleic	0	0	0.78	4.2	0.3	2.7	5.7
C18:1	Oleic	5.8	11.4	16.2	36.0	36.6	0	37.3
C18:1t	Elaidic*	0	0	2.42	0	0	0	0
C18:1t	Vaccenic*	0	0	0	0	0	0	0
C20:1	Gadoleic	0	0	0.08	0.3	0.1	1.0	1.1
C22:1	Erucic	0	0	0	0	0	0	0
C18:2	Linoleic	1.8	1.6	2.21	3.1	9.1	10.2	19.5
C18:3	Linolenic	0	0	0.25	0.6	0	0.1	1.0
C18:3	α-Linolenic	0	0	0	0	0.2	0	0
C18:4	Moroctic	0	0	0	0	0	0	0
C20:4	Arachidonic	0	0	0	0	0	0	0.1
C20:5	EPA	0	0	0	0	0	0	0
C22:5	DPA	0	0	0	0	0	0	0
C22:6	DHA	0	0	0	0	0	0	0
	PUFA	1.8	1.6	2.46	3.7	9.3	10.3	20.5
	PI	1.9	1.9	4.8	5.3	10.4	13.3	23.0
	Source	[174]	[175]	[176]	[177]	[178]	[179]	[180]

Table 15-5. Continued

Chain Length: Double Bonds	Fatty Acid	Olive oil	Canola oil	Corn oil	Soy bean oil	Cod liver oil	Krill oil
C4:0	Butyric	0	0	0	0	0	0
C6:0	Caproic	0	0	0	0	0	0
C8:0	Caprylic	0	0	0	0	0	0
C10:0	Capric	0	0	0	0	0	0
C12:0	Lauric	0	0	0	0	0	0
C14:0	Myristic	0	0	0.02	0	3.57	2.33
C16:0	Palmitic	11.3	4.3	10.6	10.45	10.63	12.56
C17:0	Margaric	0	0.05	0.07	0.03	0	0.17
C18:0	Stearic	1.95	2.09	1.85	4.44	2.8	2.39
C20:0	Arachidic	0	0	0	0	0	0.25
C22:0	Behenic	0	0.34	0.27	0.37	0	0
C16:1	Palmitoleic	1.25	0.21	0.11	0	8.31	2.19
C18:1	Oleic	71.3	61.75	27.3	22.55	20.65	7.89
C18:1t	Elaidic*	0	0.29	0	0	0	0
C18:1t	Vaccenic*	0	0	0	0	0	4.3
C20:1	Gadoleic	0.31	1.08	0.13	0.23	10.42	1.01
C22:1	Erucic	0	0	0	0	7.33	0.72
C18:2	Linoleic	9.76	18.64	53.6	50.42	0.94	1.57
C18:3	Linolenic	0	0	0	0	0.93	0.96
C18:3	α-Linolenic	0.76	9.14	1.61	6.79	0	0
C18:4	Moroctic	0	0	0	0	0.93	1.78
C20:4	Arachidonic	0	0	0	0	0.93	1.4
C20:5	EPA	0	0	0	0	6.9	31.92
C22:5	DPA	0	0	0	0	0.93	3.07
C22:6	DHA	0	0	0	0	10.97	20.53
	PUFA	10.5	28.1	54.7	57.7	22.5	59.5
	PI	13.1	38.5	56.6	64.6	146.2	397.3
	Source	[181]	[182]	[183]	[184]	[185]	[186]

MONOUNSATURATED FATS in Table 15-5 are mostly represented with the oleic (C18:1) acid with its highest content in olive (71.3%) and canola (61.7%) oils. Although both these oils are touted as "heart-healthy," as was shown earlier, their propensity to oxidation results in less than healthy outcomes [86, 87, 144]. Other oils high in oleic acid are safflower (74.6%), macadamia nut (67.1%), and sunflower (57.0%) oils.

Of the polyunsaturated PUFA fats in Table 15-5, linoleic acid (C18:2) is most abundant in corn (53.6%) and soybean (50.4%) oils. Some other vegetable oils with an even higher content of linoleic acid are: evening primrose (75.1%), grape seed (69.6%), and hemp seed (55.5%) oils. Linoleic acid has two double bonds subject to oxygen attacks, and oils containing it become easily rancid and exert many deleterious effects on health. First comes its immunosuppressive action, which weakens our defenses against viral and bacterial infections and opens the door to cancer development.

Each of the fatty acids is metabolized differently and has a specific physiological function depending on the carbon chain length and a number of double bonds. The health benefits of some saturated fatty acids were discussed earlier. We can see from Table 15-5 that butter is the only exogenous (coming from outside) source of the short-chain butyric acid which is mostly produced endogenously in our intestines by the fermentation of fiber in food. Other food sources include cream and ghee that is made from butter by simmering. In 100 g of butter, fat content is 81.1 g and 17.9 g of water is also present, thus ghee which is devoid of water has even more butyric acid.

Medium-Chain Triglycerides (MCTs) (C6:0 caproic through C12:0 lauric acid) are the most abundant in coconut (59.6%) and palm kernel (54.2%) oils and in a smaller amount (6.7%) in butter. These saturated MCT oils are metabolized more easily than long-chain fats and are used as an immediate source of energy rather than deposited in adipose tissue. This feature gained them popularity in weight loss programs. In a study of 31 subjects aged 19 to 50 years for 16 weeks, those taking 18 to 24 g/day of MCT oil lost 3.2 kg of body weight, but controls that consumed the same amount of olive oil lost only 1.4 kg [230].

In another randomized, double-blind, clinical trial on 40 Brazilian women aged 20 to 40 years with abdominal obesity, researchers investigated the effect of coconut oil on waist circumferences and cholesterol profiles. Both groups of 20 women each were supplemented with 30 mL of either coconut oil (Group C) or soybean oil (Group S) for 12 weeks.

In the coconut oil group, a reduction of waist circumferences were observed, but no changes were documented in the soybean oil group. HDL (good) cholesterol of 48.7 was higher in Group C than in Group S (45.0), and the LDL/HDL ratio was lower in Group C (2.41 vs. 3.1). From these ratios, I calculated that LDL cholesterol actually went lower in Group C (117.8) than in Group S (139.5) [231].

In this study, the coconut oil with its 93.4% saturated fat and 1.8% PUFA reduced, not raised LDL (bad) cholesterol level. Soybean oil composed of 15.6% saturated fat and 57.7% PUFA was no match for coconut oil in reducing LDL. Viva Coco, you won!

Now, if we extend best wishes to and say goodbye to the Creole beauties, who became a bit slimmer eating coconut oil, and take a flight from sunny Rio to foggy London, we will be rewarded upon arrival with another coco surprise. Coconut oil reduced LDL concentrations here too. In a randomized trial of 80 healthy men and women aged 50-75 years, divided into three groups, each subject received either 50 g of extra virgin coconut oil or of extra virgin olive oil or of unsalted butter in addition to their usual diets for 4 weeks. The mean LDL cholesterol in the butter group increased by 12.8 mg/dl (0.33 mmol/L), but decreased in the olive and coconut oil groups by 2.3 mg/dl (0.06 mmol/L) and 3.5 mg/dl (0.09 mmol/L) respectively.

The highly saturated coconut oil performed in this trial even better than the "heart-healthy" monounsaturated olive oil. Quite importantly, the levels of C-reactive protein, an indicator of inflammation and a better than LDL predictor of cardiovascular risk [232] went up by 0.23 mg/L in the olive oil group and went down by 0.31 mg/L and 0.04 mg/L in coconut oil and butter groups, respectively[189]. In other words, olive oil displayed pro inflammatory, but coconut oil and butter anti-inflammatory effects. Again, coconut oil in this respect too was superior in all three tested fats.

In England we will say hello to Zoë Harcombe, an Albion beauty and obesity researcher who advocates real food and wants us to stop eating processed foods [233]. As they do not generally grow coconuts in England, they have to import them. If we want to look at the populations where coconuts are a mainstay in their diets then we need to fly (literally or in our imagination) to the Polynesian atolls of Tokelau, Kitawa and Pukapuka in the South Pacific. These people are noted for their high consumption of saturated fats which come from coconuts rather than animal sources. In Tokelau, about half of their calorie intake is derived from saturated fat, the highest proportion recorded in the world.

The main source of their carbohydrates are tubers such as yam, sweet potato, taro, and fruit. They eat some fish but tropical fish is low in PUFAs and hence less deleterious to health than cold water fish. The common denominator for the people in these islands is that their diets are based on real foods and have very small amounts of Western processed foods. As a result, these tropical paradise dwellers enjoy good health and have very low rates of heart diseases, cancer, and diabetes [234].

On our travels there our next stop will be Kerala, India where coconut oil is a staple in cooking [235].

In my favorite Italian movie, *The Orientals (Le Orientali)*, a girl rides a bicycle along the sea coast in Malaysia and arrives at a coconut grove. She beguiles the owner with her beauty and charm and receives eight free coconuts. A little monkey with strong arms that was sitting in the girl's bicycle basket, her companion, climbs a tall coconut tree, chooses the ripe coconuts and twists them a few times until the coconut falls down on the grass.

After all eight coconuts are dropped, the girl commands the monkey to descend. Upon returning home, a family member opens one of the coconuts and gives it to the monkey to drink its milk, A "perfect symbiosis"— the monkey is not paid by the day, but is rewarded by being engaged in a "social contract," the movie's narrator comments.

On my cruise to Australia, we stopped at American Samoa and I had a chat with Bruce, an American. He married a local noblewoman and has lived there since 1980. He said his grandmother taught him to cook only with coconut oil. On our next stop at Dravuni Island, Fiji, with only a hundred or so inhabitants living off the grid, I bought a coconut on the shore from a local guy who opened it with a machete. Then I drank its water and ate a jelly scraped from the inside with a spoon. The palm trees were not as tall as in Malaysia, and there were no monkeys in sight, so another guy used a long bamboo pole to drop the coconut from the tree.

Is canola oil used for cooking on cruise ships free of *trans* fats?

Every guest of the Holland America Line cruises receives a daily program, which has a footer named, "Did you Know?" One such footer reads, "Holland America Line is committed to serving high quality, delicious, and healthy food. For that reason, we do not cook any of our foods with oils containing artificial ***trans* fats** and are proud to say that we have not done so since 2005."

"Well, well, well," as James 'Sawyer,' a character in the *'Lost'* TV show, would have said. I did two 21 day cruises with Holland America Line, one from Los Angeles to Sydney, Australia on the ship named *Volendam* in September–October 2014 and another one, a Caribbean and Central America cruise from Tampa, Florida on its ship the *Ryndam* in January–February 2015.

On both cruises, I asked the chefs what kind of oil do they use for their cooking? The answer was, "Canola oil." For breakfast, for instance, they cook egg omelets spraying Teflon-covered fry pans with canola oil. So, at the very core of their fancy food, prepared by top international chefs and cooks, was adulterated common supermarket canola oil. The question arises, whether canola oil is healthy and free of *trans* fats, as they claim or not. And here begins our canola oil adventure.

It is commonplace in the field of nutrition that food producers and consumers are on opposing sides and are in a state of continuous conflict. And the canola oil case is not an exception.

In the New York Times article, *"A Dangerous Fat and Its Risky*

Alternative" published on October 10, 2006 the author Michael Mason reflects the conventional wisdom saying, "...the saturated fats that have long been high on the list of artery-clogging foods," and "...tropical oils, like palm oil and coconut oil, or butter. Loaded with artery-blocking saturated fat..," and finally he states, "Better saturated fat, the heart-stopping devil you know? Or trans fat, the heart-stopping devil you've just been introduced to?" [236].

Alice H. Lichtenstein, one public health policy maker, was quoted as saying, "Anything was good if it decreased saturated fat consumption in the 1950s through the 1980s. But then studies began to question trans fats." The author of the article explains, "When vegetable oil is turned into a solid, like butter, it acts like butter inside the body. Trans fats were developed during the backlash against saturated fat —the artery-clogging animal fats found in butter, cream, and meats" [237].

Interestingly, industrially produced *trans* fats in hydrogenated vegetable oil are erroneously equated in this article to those found in butter, cream, and meats, which are "ruminant *trans* fats" that happened to be benign in the artery-clogging business [238] It is so typical to call saturated fat, "artery-clogging or artery-blocking," as if it is a well established and unquestioned fact. Turns out, it is not [239]. If they and their kin only knew... 'Sawyer,' where are you with your, 'Well, well, well' retort?

As the NHS, HPFS, PREDIMED and other observational studies do not distinguish between Blood types, they do not distinguish between the action of nutrients in **healthy and diseased** people as well. The authors of the NHS and the HPFS studies claim that saturated and *trans* fats were harmful but unsaturated (MUFAs and PUFAs) were beneficial to the medical professionals. However, the toxicity of fatty acids increases exponentially with their increasing degree of unsaturation expressed by the peroxidability index PI [240].

Is it possible that participants of these long-term studies had developed heart disease, cancer, etc. eating toxic unsaturated and *trans* fats in the first place, but after their disease had been established, they started to either benefit from them and survived (Blood type O, B, A2) or continued to be harmed and eventually died (Blood type AB, A1)?

In other words, poison killed the weakest, but after doing some harm turned into a healing agent for the stronger ones.

We can try to apply this alternative explanation with established heart disease to the clinical trials like the Lyon Diet Heart Study conducted in 1988-1992 in France. This clinical parallel, randomized, single-blinded trial of 605 subjects (91% men) with a median age of 53.5 years, who had survived a myocardial infarction (heart attack), was designed to test whether a diet higher in vegetable oils and lower in butter could reduce a second heart attack and death.

The experimental group of 302 patients was advised to follow a Mediterranean-type diet that contained more whole-grain bread, more green and root vegetables, olive oil and rapeseed oil for salads, more fish and poultry and less red meat, fruit every day, and a special margarine made of rapeseed oil in place of cream and butter. The control group of 303 patients continued to eat their usual French "prudent" diet advised by their doctors and dietitians. The composition of the experimental and control diets is shown in Table 15-6.

Within two years of the trial, there were 6 cardiac and 8 non-cardiac deaths in the intervention group and 19 cardiac and 5 non-cardiac deaths in the control group. The list of risk factors considered in this trial included diet, age, gender, smoking, total and HDL cholesterol, blood pressure, blood glucose, serum albumin, and leukocyte and neutrophil counts. Unfortunately, the list did not include blood type, blood viscosity [241], blood coagulation factors, e.g. von Willebrand factor and Factor VIII (both factors 25 % lower in Blood type O people than in non-Os) [242], personality type [243], overindulgence in sex [244], stress level [245] and body height [246], which makes this trial hard to interpret.

The causal factor of fewer deaths and non-fatal heart events, emphasized by authors, is a much higher (0.81 E% vs 0.27 E%) content of α-linolenic acid (C18:3, ω-3 or n-3) in the experimental group (Table 15-6). We can look at α-linolenic acid as a deleterious agent in the development of heart disease before myocardial infarction (in health), and serves as a curative agent after myocardial infarction (in disease). α-linolenic acid is synthesized in plants. e.g. seeds, nuts, grain, or grass and serves as fuel for germination, hence the germ of grain, seeds, and nuts has a higher content than the remainder. The colder the temperature of the soil in spring, the higher the concentration of α-linolenic acid in the seed, which makes oil more liquid, prevents the seeds from freezing and ensures germination and propagation of the plants.

Table 15-6. Composition of Experimental & Control Diets

Entry	Experimental Diet	Control Diet	Ratio Experim/ Control. %
Energy, kcal	1928	2140	90.1
Carbohydrates, % energy	52.3	50.8	102.9
Protein, % energy	17.2	16.5	104.2
Total fat, % energy	30.5	32.7	93.3
Butter and cream, g/day	2.8	16.6	16.9
Margarine, g/day	19.0	5.1	372.5
Saturated fat, % energy	8.3	11.7	70.9
Oleic acid, % energy	12.9	10.3	125.2
Linoleic acid, % energy	3.6	5.3	67.9
α-linolenic acid, % energy	0.81	0.27	300
Trans fat, % energy	5.4	1.4*	385.7
Total Cholesterol, mg/dl	217	318	68.2
Fiber, g	18.6	15.5	120
Lipid lowering drugs, %	26.5	34.0	77.9

* Estimated in proportion to the margarine content.

The plants that grow in northern climates such as flax seeds or high in the mountains such as chia (7.4%) in the Andes mountains contain more α-linolenic acid than tropical plants, (e.g. coconuts or safflower seeds) that contain zero. Thus, latitude and altitude of the region where plants grow determine their α-linolenic acid content. The same applies to linolenic acid (C18:3) in algae, fish or seafood: Alaskan salmon contains more linolenic acid than tropical fish. In its α-linolenic acid concentration, grass is also different according to the latitude or altitude of its growing area. Among other benefits, the higher content of α-linolenic acid in grass-fed beef is considered to make it superior in nutritional quality than the grain-fed.

I wonder, how latitude or altitude of the pasture where the cows graze would influence the beef's linolenic acid content. α-linolenic acid (C18:3) is a long-chain polyunsaturated fatty acid PUFA with three double bonds which are the sites of instability and are subject to oxygen attack. The hydrogen atom adjacent to the double bond has a weak adherence to the carbon atom, which makes it easy to be displaced from its position. As soon as α-linolenic acid is formed in the maturing seed, nut, grain [72] or grass, its double bonds become a target for an attack from Reactive Oxygen Species (ROS).

ROS being "the uninvited companions of aerobic life" which are produced continuously as byproducts of metabolism in different plant cell organelles such as chloroplasts, mitochondria, and peroxisomes. ROS, e.g. superoxide, hydroxyl, perhydroxy and alkoxy radicals, hydrogen peroxide and singlet oxygen, "are highly reactive and toxic and cause damage to proteins, carbohydrates, lipids, and DNA which ultimately results in cell death" [247].

One of the most damaging effects of ROS is the peroxidation of lipids that creates lipid hydroperoxides. They are unstable compounds and "can easily decompose into several reactive species: lipid alkoxyl radicals, aldehydes (malonyldialdehyde), alkanes, lipid epoxides, and alcohols" [248]. The removal of a hydrogen atom from the carbon atom next to the double bond initiates a cascade of reactions. The first stage of oxidation is called autoxidation and takes place in the absence of air, inside of the air-tight nut or seed shell, e.g. in almonds, sunflower or flax seeds. Naturally occurring antioxidants in the oil, such as tocopherols block these free radicals and temporarily hinder the progression of the free radical chain reaction. After antioxidants are used up, seeds age more rapidly.

Seeds, nuts, grains, and grass grow and mature in an oxygen-rich environment and oxygen, as a major free radical, being exposed to light generates singlet oxygen that interacts with double bonds. This process is called photo-oxidation and proceeds 30,000 times faster than auto-oxidation [247]. Yet another mechanism of oxidation known as the enzymatic peroxidation occurs under the action of enzymes that are present in plants, e.g. lipoxygenase and cyclooxygenase, which catalyze reactions between oxygen and PUFA double bonds [249]. Lipid peroxidation is also enhanced by high temperature and metal catalysts, e.g. iron and copper.

Lipid peroxidation of linoleic acid (C18:2) produces a toxic alde-hyde, 4-hydroxy-2-nonenal (HNE) and that of α-linolenic acid (C18:3) – 4-hydroxy-2-hexenal (HHE) [250]. A secondary peroxidation prod-uct, malondialdehyde (MDA) is formed from both linoleic and α-linolenic acids.

After seeds, grains and nuts are harvested, their storage leads to further degradation of PUFAs, loss of fatty acids and increased produc-tion of HNE and MDA. High humidity storage for 6 days resulted in a marked loss of linoleic (C18:2) and α-linolenic acid (C18:3) in the phospholipid fraction of the "soybean axis" from an initial 57.3% and 19.3% to 33.9% and 6.5%, respectively [251]. At the same time, MDA levels significantly increased. Low storage humidity did not exert such degradation.

An extraction of oils from seeds, nuts or fish, which involves more exposure to oxygen, usually performed under the elevated temperatures (even cold-pressed) and with the use of chemical solvents, further decomposes fatty acids and produces more HNE and MDA [252]. As we discussed before, the oil in living fish is protected against oxidation in its water habitat, but as soon as it is taken into the air, it begins to oxidize. The extraction of fish oil speeds up this process. Purification and deodorization of oils under high temperature and more chemical solvents, e.g. hexane, creates *trans* fats [253].

As if that were not enough, cooking and deep frying in vegetable oils for hours generates more peroxidation compounds that are incor-porated into foods, such as fried chicken, donuts, potato chips, and French fries. The level of HNE, although undetected before heating, was greatly increased "in soybean oil that was heated at 185°C for 2, 4,

6, 8, and 10 h" [254]. It sounds doubtful to me, though, that no HNE was found in this study in the soybean oil before cooking.

In another study, "Dietary oils—tuna, salmon, cod liver, soybean, olive, and corn oils—were treated with accelerated storage conditions (60 degrees C for 3 and 7 d) and a cooking condition (200 degrees C for 1 h)." "Salmon oil produced the greatest amount of MA (1070+/-77.0 ppm of oil) when it was heated at 60 degrees C for 7 d" [254]. In this study, MA is referring to malondialdehyde which is usually abbreviated as MDA. "When oils were treated under cooking conditions, the aldehydes formed were comparable to those formed under accelerated storage conditions" [255].

It means that the amount of MDA generated during one hour of cooking at the temperature of 200 °C or 392 °F was about the same as formed in 7 days of storage temperature at 60 °C or 140 °F. I doubt that **the Japanese authors** of this study when they saw firsthand how deleterious to health is **deep frying in oils at high temperatures** will ever touch tempura again, a popular Japanese dish of seafood fried in oil. During my five years in Japan, I ate my share of tempura. If I only knew!

These multi-stage processes from maturing of seeds or nuts to their storage to the extraction of oil to oil storage and oil heating in cooking produce increasing amounts of exogenous toxic aldehydes, but once inside our body, under the process of normal metabolism, yet additional endogenous HNE and MDA are generated [256]. These toxic compounds are absorbed into the blood and tissues and cause endothelial injury, which can overwhelm our immune system and cause inflammation in various organs.

Acute inflammation activates the immune system in response to viral or bacterial infection, irritation, or injury. The number of white blood cells is increased and redness, hotness, swelling and pain of the tissues manifest. If this normal response of the system to irritation or injury persists, it turns into chronic inflammation, which "underlay a variety of human diseases, including cardiovascular disease, cancer, diabetes and neurodegenerative disease" [257, p.134]. Chronic inflammation due to the endothelium (blood vessel wall) injury is believed to be an underlying cause of atherosclerosis leading to heart attacks and stroke [258].

We saw how harmful wrong fats could be to our health. Other macronutrients in our food, e.g. carbohydrates and proteins, although necessary for the proper functioning of our system, impose their own deleterious effects if consumed in excess or of the wrong kind.

11

HOW ESSENTIAL ARE CARBOHYDRATES?

Carbohydrates are organic compounds of carbon, hydrogen, and oxygen (hence their name), which are represented mainly by sugar and starch. Broken down by digestion into glucose, fructose, and galactose (milk sugar), they circulate in the blood and are delivered to cells where they are metabolized to provide our body with energy for rapid use. End products of their metabolism are carbon dioxide and metabolic water.

Carbohydrates are virtually all of plant origin, although they also are present in milk. They are divided into two categories: simple (refined) carbohydrates or sugars, and complex carbohydrates. *Simple carbohydrates* are abundant in white bread, white pasta, white rice, sugary cereals and snacks, cookies, and cakes. Plant sources of sugars include sugar beets, sugar cane, fruits and honey. *Complex carbohydrates* come from fruits and vegetables, whole grains, breads, pastas, cereals, and legumes.

Health experts and policymakers in nutrition maintain that carbohydrates are good for our health and longevity and the best ones are complex carbohydrates. Some experts even call complex carbohydrates life-extenders, because they largely exist in the diet in the world's "blue zones" of longevity.

Fruits are always on the top of their list, and they are even called rejuvenating carbohydrates, followed by vegetables. However, sugars and starchy vegetables such as potatoes and corn can cause a sudden rise in blood glucose, which has a detrimental effect on our health and are reputed to be age accelerators. Any carbohydrates eaten in excess leads to weight gain; therefore, weight-reducing high-protein diet proponents fight an unceasing war against them.

Carbohydrates, which are the most prevalent macronutrient for a majority of the world population, when eaten bring about our body's response by the secretion of hormones (growth factors) such as insulin and Insulin-like Growth Factors IGF 1 and IGF 2. The secretion of insulin in our pancreas, expressed as an Insulin Score (IS), depends on the glycemic index and the glycemic load induced by carbohydrates and is discussed in Chapter 10 of my book, "Control for Life ...." [259].

These growth factors, including insulin, prompt our cells to grow and proliferate, which are not necessary after we have grown up and become adults. And even very dangerous if the new cells are cancerous. Rather, we need our cells to focus on maintenance and repair activities more than anything else.

Another problem with carbohydrates is that their derivatives, reducing sugars such as glucose, fructose, galactose (milk sugar), lactose, and maltose (malt sugar) react with amino acids binding to them and thus impairing their normal function. Dark-color products are formed and the process is called *non-enzymic glycosylation (glycation),* known also as the browning effect or Millard reaction.

The browning effect is observed in the crust of bread or pizza, in glazed meat, baked or roasted vegetables when high temperatures are used in cooking. It enhances the palatability of food and is welcomed in the culinary arts; however, it has a side effect since, upon oxidation, it creates advanced glycation end products (AGEs). In AGEs, "the protein molecules are basically glued together in an irreversible way that stiffens and degrades them" [150, p.40].

A similar process occurs inside our body when the circulating glucose in our blood derived from sugar and starch of the carbohy-drates is not used for immediate energy. The major function of insulin is to deliver glucose or other sugars to cells where they are metabolized for energy and thus clearing the blood of glucose. If cells resist taking up glucose (known as insulin resistance, but actually glucose resistance) and glucose concentration in the blood becomes elevated, then AGEs are formed endogenously. AGEs are found to adversely affect many of our physiological functions.

One of the examples is thickening and decreased permeability in the *basement membrane*, a coating over endothelial cells of the capillaries. This impairs capillary exchange: infusion of oxygen and nutrients from the blood into the interstitial liquid and further into cells and collection of carbon dioxide and the end products of cell metabolism into the blood for elimination.

Another example is the stiffening of collagen tissue in tendons, blood vessels and joints [116, p.230]. Yet one more example is glucose binding to hemoglobin, a principal protein of red blood cells, forming glycated (glycosylated) hemoglobin HbA1c, which is a good indicator of how much one's system is affected by blood glucose.

The more glucose that circulates in the blood, the more hemoglobin becomes glycated and the higher the HbA1c value is. The normal (non-diabetic) value of HbA1c is 6% which corresponds to a blood glucose level of 120 mg/dl [260, p.116]. People with diabetes have levels of HbA1c higher than that.

The adverse effects of elevated blood glucose were found to be linked to increased mortality in a study of 2501 men and women aged 65 years or older in four US communities. In this prospective population-based cohort study conducted in 1989-1990, 646 deaths were recorded within five years of follow up. Among 20 characteristics, "significantly and independently associated with mortality" were increasing age, male sex, low body weight, and "elevated fasting glucose level (>7.2 mmol/L [130 mg/dL])," just to name a few [261].

Notably, total, HDL or LDL cholesterols showed no association with mortality. More than that, "...LDL cholesterol level higher than 3.96 mmol/L (153 mg/dL) had a significantly lower risk (RR, 0.66), compared with lower values of LDL cholesterol" [261]. This is another nail in the "lower-your-cholesterol" policy coffin.

No matter how many nails are in the cholesterol coffin, both coffin and the cholesterol myth seem to coexist in parallel. The cholesterol hysteria still sells to millions. All the studies (discussed in Chapter 5 of this book) on deadly effects of low cholesterol levels seem to be unknown to (or ignored by) Michael Greger, MD, a leading author of the New York Times bestselling book, *How Not To Die: Discover the Foods Scientifically Proven to Prevent and Reverse Disease.*

In the chapter, *How Not To Die from Heart Disease,* Dr. Greger's prescription is simple and crystal clear—lower your cholesterol. He claims support from the insights of William C. Roberts, MD, the editor in chief of the *American Journal of Cardiology* for over 30 years, who "has authored more than a thousand scientific publications and written more than a dozen textbooks on cardiology. He knows his stuff" [262, p.32]. He invites us to trust Dr. Roberts who 'knows his stuff' as much as he does himself.

Dr. Roberts states that "the only critical risk factor for atherosclerotic plaque buildup is cholesterol, specifically elevated LDL cholesterol in your blood" [262, p.32]. Roberts expressed this critical statement on the cause of heart disease in his editorial article, *It's the Cholesterol, Stupid!* "The lower the LDL cholesterol the better, and this principle has been established repeatedly despite the voices of the anticholesterol, antistatin fallacy mongers! It's the cholesterol, stupid!" [263]. Dr. Greger seems to get a kick out of this phrase and has it in bold font as a heading of the subsection in his chapter.

Dr. Roberts explains where this phrase came from, "During the 1992 presidential campaign in the USA, the Clinton campaign the slogan was "It's the economy, stupid," and that phrase apparently was helpful in getting Mr. Clinton elected president" [263]. In a similar manner, Drs. Roberts and Greger rely on the magic power of this slogan and don't bother to give extensive supporting evidence.

Dr Greger indicates the causes of the "number-one killer," which are "...the trans fat, saturated fat, and cholesterol-laden foods that clog our arteries" [262, p.30]. He confines his supporting evidence to mentioning two populations: the rural Guizhou province of China (half million people) and Uganda, "a country of millions in eastern Africa" where heart disease is extremely rare. The common thread in these two cultures is a plant-based diet that is low in animal foods and cholesterol [262, p.29]. He fails to mention, though, the studies of Masai people in Africa by George Mann, MD, and dwellers of the Polynesian atolls of Tokelau, Kitawa, and Pukapuka in the South Pacific [234] and Kerala in India [235] who did not have heart disease on animal-based or very high saturated fat diets.

Dr. Mann studied 1,500 Masai, the "East African tribesmen who subsist almost solely on their cattle, consuming meat, blood and milk." He found that "they have very low levels of cholesterol in their blood, half as much as we do, and very rarely have cardiovascular disease" [264].

Dr. Mann and his colleagues investigated the condition of the heart and blood vessels of 50 Masai men that were collected at autopsy. Milk and meat predominate in the diet of these people and their "intake of animal fat exceeds that of American men." Although their aortas showed "extensive atherosclerosis with lipid infiltration and fibrous changes, but very few complicated lesions" were documented. The intimal thickening of the coronary arteries by atherosclerosis was present as much as that in U.S. elderly men. The researchers stated that the blood vessels of Masai people "enlarge with age to more than compensate for this disease." Their conclusion reads, "It is speculated that the Masai are protected from their atherosclerosis by physical fitness which causes their coronary vessels to be capacious" [265]. In other words, Masai people have atherosclerosis but don't suffer from heart disease. It would be a conundrum for Drs. Roberts, Greger and their vegetarian kin.

Dr. Greger could also mention a study of 94 Japanese centenarians and 422 city residents aged 69-71 who consumed more "animal foods such as eggs, milk, fish and meat" and fewer carbohydrates than their average fellow Japanese [266]. Or a study of Okinawans who eat pork and poultry [52 p.73] and have the highest ratio of centenarians of any nation.

In the ever-lasting diet wars, it is not unusual to accuse an opponent of being 'wrong' on all counts as Dr. Dean Ornish in the past did in a debate with Dr. Robert Atkins [267], or more recently, Nina Teicholz in a dispute with Dr. Ornish [268]. Dr. Greger does the same stating *The Plant Paradox* (Dr. Gundry) [269] or Blood type diet (Dr. D'Adamo) [270] are all wrong. Teicholz is involved again and calls Dr. Greger "a radical animal welfare activist" who advocates not eating animal foods for ethical reason. She adds, "so this is his agenda, not nutrition" [271].

Although I disagree with Dr. Greger on fundamental issues such as effects of saturated fat, cholesterol, lectins abundant in his legumes and grains and the Blood type connection and consider his vegan diet extreme and harmful in the long run, there are few points in his book that are appealing to me:

1. the inefficacy of omega-3 supplements to improve hearth health [262, p.30];

2. the danger of statin drugs [262, p.33].

The negative side effects of omega-3 intake for our health are extensively discussed in this book. The heart disease and omega-3 connection was investigated in the study of 130 Greenland Eskimos, 32 Greenland Eskimos living in Denmark and of 31 Caucasian Danes in Denmark byDyerberg, Bang, and Hjorne. The diet of native Greenland Eskimos was rich in whale meat and seal blubber. The researchers found that the "total concentration of polyunsaturated fatty acids was lower in Greenland Eskimos than in the other groups." Also they noted that "...coronary atherosclerosis seems to occur far less commonly among Eskimos in Greenland than among peoples in industrialized countries..." [272].

It seems that the lower the PUFA levels in the blood, the better it is for heart health. The notion of Dyerberg, et al. about low rates of atherosclerosis and coronary artery disease among Greenland Eskimos had been widely accepted as an established fact. As a consequence, this study had a big impact on the official dietary recommendation to increase intake of cold-water fish and omega-3 supplements for a healthy heart. However, later it was found that Greenland Eskimos suffered from heart disease at the same rate and their stroke mortality was even higher than among their Denmark counterparts [273].

As a serious researcher who prefers searching for scientific papers

(100,000 a year) [269] rather than being engaged in the "diet wars," why would Dr. Greger bother himself to present a piece of evidence supporting the opposite of his thesis. It is not his business, it is a business of his critics. His mentor (Dr. Roberts) didn't do that and the mentor of his mentor (Dr. Keys) didn't do that either. Their strongest ploy was to call people 'stupid' or 'monger' and that was good enough.

Dr. Greger asserts, those who have heart disease can reverse it by following a low fat, plant-based diet, the core of the Nathan Pritikin, Dean Ornish and Caldwell Esselstyn Jr. protocols [262, p.34]. These vegetarian devotees seem to be role models for Dr. Greger, but are they for us too?

Nathan Pritikin (1915-1985), a founder of Pritikin Longevity Center, suffered from leukemia, underwent chemotherapy treatment for two years without success and committed suicide at the age of 69 and half years. No signs of atherosclerosis were found at his autopsy [274]. Whether it was the result of his low-fat diet or his illness remains unclear.

Dean Ornish, 65, MD was criticized that it is uncertain whether 41 patients in his study improved their cardiovascular health because of his low fat diet alone or the combined effect of diet, yoga, exercise, social supports, or dietary supplements that were part of his intervention. His critics also point out that to prove his beliefs he cites epidemiological (observational) and mice studies which are considered irrelevant [268].

Caldwell Esselstyn Jr., 85, MD faces a similar criticism of his even smaller (18 patients) than Ornish's (41 patients) study based on a dietary questionnaire which his patients filled out. That kind of study is considered unreliable. In the article, "The incredibly bad science behind Dr. Esselstyn's plant-based diet," the 'skeptical cardiologist' points out that patients were on cholesterol-lowering drugs, there was no control group and in the study group "Three of the 18 patients have died, one from pulmonary fibrosis, one presumably from a GI bleed, and one from depression" [275]. From the initial group of 24 patients, six patients dropped out being unable to comply with his fat-stringent diet (even no avocados or olive oil). One must be very motivated to continue this diet which is unsustainable for most people long-term.

Also, it occurs that coronary artery blockage is not the only cause of heart disease. In his book, *Prevent and Reverse Heart Disease*, Dr. Esselstyn shows three drawings of the gradual build-up of plaque inside a coronary artery and the closing of the lumen (vessel inner channel). In the last of these three artery cross-sections, plaque fills the whole cross-section with only a tiny hole close to the center available for blood flow. The drawing description reads, "Figure 2. Gradually progressive coronary artery narrowing, which accounts for 12.5 percent of heart attacks" [170, color insert following p.116].

It means that only one in eight heart attacks is caused by artery occlusion (stenosis). The majority, or seven in eight heart attacks are attributed to lactic acid buildup in heart muscles caused by physical or emotional stress and the predominance of the Sympathetic Nervous System syndrome, discussed in my book, "*Why Women Live Longer and What Men Can Do About It.*" It looks like Dr. Greger's claims are supported by giants with feet of clay.

Dr. Roberts, the ultimate authority on heart disease for Dr. Greger, in his turn claims support from the Seven Countries Study by Ancel Keys and Co. that was refuted in more than one serious analysis [98, 133, 141, 233, 361]. His other supporting argument that "elevated cholesterol" causes atherosclerosis is that "Atherosclerotic plaques are easily produced experimentally in herbivores (e.g., rabbits, monkeys) simply by feeding these animals cholesterol (e.g., egg yokes) or saturated fats" and "it is not possible to produce atherosclerosis in carnivores (dogs, cats, tigers, lions, etc)" [263].

The question arises now, we humans, are we herbivores or carnivores? The definitive answer can be found when we look at the acidity of our digestive juices or stomach acid. On the continuous scale of the stomach PH values (acidity-alkalinity) for birds and mammals, the obligate scavengers (vulture, turkey) have the lowest PH of 1.3, followed by PH of 1.8 for facultative scavengers (red-tailed hawk), and then PH of 2.2 for generalist carnivore (chicken). In the middle of the scale is omnivore (adult human) with PH of 2.9 followed by specialist carnivore (insectivorous bat) with PH of 3.6. On the high end of the scale are hind-gut herbivores (African elephant) with PH of 4.1 and finally foregut herbivores (colobus monkey) with PH of 6.1.

Notably, humans are omnivores and evolved eating animal flesh (raw fish, raw mammal meat) [276]. In some cultures like Japan, sushi and sashimi (raw fish) or raw caribou (reindeer) meat among Alaskan Inuits is a common dish. It looks like the vegan gurus including Drs. Rogers and Greger are on a mission to elevate human nature by converting them into herbivores.

It sounds disturbing to me but Americans seem not to mind when in popular books they are called 'idiots' (e.g.,   *TheComplete Idiot's Guide to Vegan Cooking*), 'dummies' (e.g., *Diabetes for Dummies*), or 'stupid' (e.g.,*Idiot America: How Stupidity Became a Virtue in the Land of the Free*) and in the above-mentioned editorial article.

People these days are so busy looking at their smartphones and texting to their friends that there is no time left in their busy schedule to notice a plain and obvious insult. The most striking case of addiction to a smartphone I witnessed at one funeral. When a girl stepped forward to say farewell to her beloved grandmother laying in the casket, her boyfriend followed her while looking at his smartphone. I imagine how disappointed these people will become when they don't find smartphones in the "better world." Well, with the advances in technology, this could become a possibility. As a contemporary Russian joke goes, there was a request to the coffin makers from oligarchs (filthy rich) to manufacture caskets with pockets so, when they died, they could take the billions of dollars stolen from the people's economy to the other side.

Dr. Greger's diet contains 1365 kcal, of which carbohydrates comprise 67.3%, protein 16.6%, and fat 16.1% [277]. It is a calorie-restricted, high-carbohydrate, low-fat diet and definitely one can lose weight on it but can they reverse diabetes too as Dr. Greger claims [262, p.133]?

A good indicator of how much one's system is affected by blood glucose is glucose binding to hemoglobin, a principal protein of red blood cells, which forms glycated (glycosylated) hemoglobin HbA1c.

Seemingly impressive results were achieved in bringing elevated HbA1c in diabetic patients down in the study of 49 subjects following a low-fat vegan diet and 50 controls following the American Diabetic Association (ADA) guidelines for 22 weeks [278]. The vegan diet consisted of grains, legumes, fruits, and vegetables, contained no animal products (resembling Dr. Greger's diet) and was a high carbo-☐ hydrate (75%), low fat (10%) and moderate protein (15%) plan. The ADA diet contained animal products but by the macronutrient struc- ture, with its protein (15-20%), saturated fat (<7%), and carbohydrates combined with monounsaturated fats (60-70%) was close to a vegan diet. The amount of mono- and polyunsaturated fats and trans fats, though, were not indicated and carbohydrates and monounsaturated fats were lumped together, which makes ADA diet's macronutrient content difficult to analyze. As a result of the study, clinical improve- ments were observed in blood glucose levels, body weight, plasma lipid concentrations, and urinary albumin excretion in both groups, but improvements were more significant in the low-fat vegan group.

Extended to 74 weeks, this study demonstrated a tendency of a gradual return to the baseline pattern in both groups. In the vegan group, the greatest HbA1c reduction of 1.23 points achieved at 22 weeks decreased to 0.82 points by 72 weeks. In the ADA group, the 0.38 figure was reduced to 0.21. This disturbing trend of continuous and not ending rebound (returning to the baseline) at 74 weeks was observed. The authors concluded that the "long-term effect of both diet interventions on glycemia was reduced in comparison with the short- term findings from this study" [279]. If prolonged even further, say for one more year, and this trend continued, possibly the benefits of a vegan diet on the HbA1c level might disappear completely. Thus, the results of these studies did not support to the claimed benefits of vegan diet.

In the chapter, *How Not to Die from Diabetes*, Dr. Greger cites a 2006 study of 22 weeks [278] but omits citing a 2009 study of 74 weeks [279], most likely because of its negative results that don't fit into his vegan agenda. Instead, he is exited describing a study that achieved great diabetes improvement not "over the course of months or years" but within 16 days [262, p.134]. The vegan gurus do it quite often, you may recall Dr. Brian Clement advocating vegetable oils and rejecting fats from animal sources. If Dr. Greger can't distinguish between short-term improvement of symptoms as opposed to the reversal of the disease, let alone its cure, than his reasoning was probably badly impaired by his extremely low-fat diet.

As was already mentioned, Dr. Greger and the proponents of a high carbohydrate diet claim that they can stop and even reverse diabetes. George L. King, MD in his book, *The Diabetes Reset: Avoid It. Control It. Even Reverse It. A Doctor's Scientific Program*, advocates "a low-fat, high-fiber diet consisting of 70% carbohydrates, 15% fat, and 15% protein, including 15 grams of dietary fiber for every 1,000 calories consumed" [280]. A promoted King's Rural Asian Diet is an exact replica of the Chinese study [281] that, like his own study, lasted only eight weeks, which is too short, as it was shown above, for his claim to be taken without a grain of salt.

Currently, ADA does not specify the amount of carbohydrate for a person with diabetes to eat. Instead, it states, "The amount of carbohydrate you need will vary based on many factors. You and your health care team can figure out the right amount for you" [282]. Dr. Mercola, the New York Times bestselling author advocates, though, the restriction of the carbohydrates, "...your best bet in managing—or even reversing—your type 2 diabetes is to adopt a low-carb, high-fat diet" [283, p.287]. This is just the opposite of what Dr. Greger and other vegan gurus recommend. A low-carbohydrate, high-fat diet, as Atkins' and Kwasniewski's diets have been discussed previously.

The Atkins diet was put to the test in a two-year-long Dietary Intervention Randomized Controlled Trial (DIRECT) in Israel. The three tested diets were: low-fat (104 participants), Mediterranean (109 participants), and Atkins, low-carbohydrate (109 participants) diet. The study revealed that "Among the participants with diabetes, the proportion of glycated hemoglobin at 24 months decreased by 0.4% in the low fat group, 0.5% in the Mediterranean-diet group, and 0.9% in the low-carbohydrate group." The weight loss, the greatest in the

Atkins diet group at 5 months, after some rebound, stabilized (reached a plateau) after 15 months [284].

Thus, the Atkins diet was the best in both HbA1c and body weight reduction. It is noteworthy that data for this study came from the food the participants actually ate which was prepared and served to them in a cafeteria, and not based on recall via a questionnaire as is the case in most studies. It is one of the most reliable studies ever, although it also has some limitations such as the absence of data on Blood type. This study also demonstrated that any nutritional intervention for diabetes shorter than 2 years must be excluded from the analysis.

12

DELETERIOUS EFFECTS OF CARBOHYDRATES

A s a consequence of undesirable effects of carbohydrates, elevated HbA1c values adversely affect our brains as well, as the Austrian Stroke Prevention Study demonstrated. It investigated annual brain volume changes in 96 females and 105 males of a median age of 60, followed for 6 years. The study found that "Glycated hemoglobin A (HbA1c) was identified as a risk factor for a greater rate of brain atrophy"[285]. Proteolitic enzymes break down undesirable glucose-protein bonds on a regular basis, but if overwhelmed, these bonds become oxidized and AGEs are formed. This process probably occurs in everybody over the years with even normal blood glucose levels but it can be faster with an increased glucose concentration, as in diabetic patients [116, p.231]. This acronym, AGEs pertains to their biological effect in aging.

The amino acids that are the most reactive to *glycation* and primary targets of AGEs are cysteine, histidine and lysine. Among carbohydrates, glucose is much less reactive than fructose but, its significantly higher concentration in the blood makes it a major player in the production of AGEs.

Carbohydrates taken in excess for prolonged periods of time increase the concentration of triglycerides in the blood through the process of a *de novo* lipogenesis. This can cause a disorder called *lipemia*, abnormal levels of fat in the blood.

Around 1955, Edward H. "Pete" Ahrens, Jr. (1915-2000), a prominent lipid researcher at Rockefeller University, called this phenomenon *"carbohydrates-induced lipemia."* "When he gave lectures, Ahrens would show photos of two test tubes of blood serum obtained from the same patient—one when the patient was eating a high-carbohydrate diet and one on a high-fat diet. One test tube would be milky white, indicating lipemia. The other would be absolutely clear" [141, p.157]. In his 1961 article, *Carbohydrate-induced and fat-induced lipemia,* Ahrens explained, "A high-fat formula was fed in one period–a fat-free, high-carbohydrate feeding in the other. It may surprise some readers to learn that the lipemic plasma was obtained during the high-carbohydrate period, and the clear plasma during the high-fat eating regimen" [286].

Although the fat-induced *lipemia* after fatty meals is a well known "physiological occurrence," over the course of a decade Ahrens observed it only in two patients, but carbohydrates-induced *lipemia*, in 13 patients. Ahrens had some evidence that the fat-induced lipemia in both cases was "a familial disorder of fat metabolism" [286]. In *de novo* lipogenesis (synthesis of fats), fatty acids and triglycerides that show up in the blood are produced mostly from a source such as glucose, "although amino acids which can be converted to acetyl-CoA can in principle also be substrates." The carbohydrate-induced *de novo* lipogenesis occurs mostly in the liver from glucose (stimulated by insulin) when all the glycogen (a storage form of glucose) deposits in the liver itself and muscles are full but there is still an excess of glucose [116, p.131-2].

In both kinds of *lipemia*, blood becomes clear of fat on a low-calorie regimen. In a 56-year-old patient, when a high-carbohydrate diet (65% to 85%) was replaced with high-fat (70%) regimen, it took four weeks for all blood lipids, e.g. total cholesterol, phospholipids and triglycerides to drop dramatically [287].

A frequent cause of *lipemia* is calorie consumption exceeding the needs of the body. Ahrens maintained that carbohydrate-induced *lipemia* does not happen in Asia and other impoverished nations where the calorie intake is low and physical activity is high. Michael Klaper, M.D., in his presentation on video, *Diet for All Reasons,* demonstrated an impressive example of *lipemia.* Dr. Klaper recounted that while working in a hospital, he was involved in the treatment of Mr. Phillip, a patient who arrived for a scheduled four-vessel coronary artery bypass surgery. Mr. Phillip's weight was 290 lb, his blood glucose level was 290, and his his systolic blood pressure and cholesterol were also 290, so Dr. Klaper nicknamed him, "Mr. Two Ninety."

Before surgery, Dr. Klaper had drawn the blood from Mr. Phillip and at a presentation, pointing at a picture of test tubes, he explained, "Here on the left, is normal serum, is normal blood. Here you see a dark red clot and this golden yellow liquid. This is a normal serum, normal blood, this is what your blood is supposed to look like. But I looked at Mr. Phillip's tube and it was so shocking. The serum flowing in his tube was thick and greasy white. It looked like almost glue, it stuck to the sides of the tube, when I shook it. I went back into the room and asked, "Mr. Phillip, did you eat before you came to the hospital?" He said, "Yes." "What did you have?" He said, "I had a double cheeseburger and a milkshake."

"And when he said that, I realized what I was looking at was all this fat in the beef burger, and butterfat in cheese, and butterfat in ice cream, and butterfat in milk, had oozed down to his bloodstream and turned his blood fatty. This well-known medical phenomenon is called *lipemia*, and it happens every time you eat a fatty meal, you turn you blood fatty. And your blood stays this way for four hours until your liver can clear it out of blood stream" [288, video 4:10-6:05]. Klaper interpreted Mr. Phillip's fatty blood as a case of *fat-induced lipemia.*

In yet another case, Keith Frayn in his 2010 edition of *Metabolic Regulation*, presented a color picture of the test tubes containing fatty blood plasma. He analyzed what happened to the blood after eating a cheese sandwich containing 50 g carbohydrates and 30 g fat. According to Frayn, carbohydrates would trigger blood glucose and insulin to rise.

Dietary fat which comes mostly in the form of triglycerides (he called them more technically, triacylglycerols) will be absorbed in the small intestines, processed by its cells to form chylomicron particles and liberated into the lymphatic system. After circulating in the lymphatic system for some time, it will enter the bloodstream. "The process is much slower than the absorption of glucose or amino acids, so that the peak in plasma triacylglycerol concentration after a fatty meal does not occur until 3-5 hours after the meal" [289, p.185].

In the tube corresponding to the cheese sandwich, the large triacyl-glycerol particles gave plasma a "milky" appearance. Clear plasma in another tube was related to the fasting state. Similar to Klaper's inter-pretation, Frayn attributed plasma turbidity to the fat in the meal ("fatty meal"). The *de novo* lipogenesis caused by the carbohydrate part of the meal was not mentioned here, although Frayn discussed this subject in different parts of his book. Perhaps, the fatty, "milky" blood in Frayn's example is limited just to the fat-induced and not attributed to carbohy-drates-induced lipogenesis because of the amount of carbohydrates in the cheese sandwich (50 g) was not that great. Mr. Phillip's case is a different story.

Using the selfnutrition.com website [290], I calculated macronutri-ents in Mr. Phillip's meal of a double cheeseburger, milkshake and ice cream (mentioned by Dr. Klaper). It contained 133 g carbohydrates, 66.4 g fat, 40.2 g protein, and 1272 kcal (64% DV), more than double amount of both carbohydrates and fat than in Frayn's example. Although Mr. Phillip's 598 cal of fat were higher than 532 cal of carbo-hydrates, of a meal total 1272 calories, they comprised 47% versus 41.5% carbohydrates or just 5.5% lower. I believe, it wouldn't be correct to totally neglect carbohydrates as a cause of   *lipemia*, as Klaper did.

Also, we need to take into account that with his 290 mg/dl blood glucose level, a grossly overweight 290 lb Mr. Phillip most likely was diabetic, had a high insulin level, and insulin resistance. Stimulated by insulin, his liver would most probably synthesize fat from an overabun-dance of glucose in his system by means of *de novo* lipogenesis.

In obese people like Mr. Phillip, the *de novo* lipogenesis on a high-carbohydrate diet was found to be up to 5-fold higher than in normal weight people [291]. Thus, most likely, Mr. Phillip's *lipemia* was not due to his rare "familial disorder of fat metabolism," but mostly carbohydrate-induced, with some contribution from fat-induced *lipemia* as well.

Dr. Klaper's appeared in the CBS documentary, *Diet for a New America: Your Health, Your Planet,* based on John Robbins' book. In this film, Robbins interviewed Dr. Klaper, John A. McDougal, M.D., and T. Colin Campbell, Ph.D., all advocates of a plant-based diet and avoidance of animal foods. Dr. Klaper's episode with Mr. Phillip's fatty test tube and his *lipemia* was shown and used as a scare tactic [292]. In that documentary, Robbins, an enthusiast and activist of vegetarian eating who had no medical or nutritional background, would explain to the audience how Mr Phillip's fatty blood would cause atherosclerosis and heart attacks. It is pretty amazing! As true crusaders of the plant-based, vegetarian movement, Robbins and Klaper emphasized the fat-containing animal food items that Mr. Phillip ate and failed to recognize the contribution of carbohydrates in that meal.

Klaper blaimed animal fat as the culprit of Mr.Phillip's clogged arteries and carbohydrates as a source of fat synthesis would not fit into his agenda. The year was 1991, and it was popular to demonize animal fat. Klaper jumped on the "animal fat is bad" bandwagon leading to a misinterpretation of Mr. Phillip's case. Sadly, Dr. Klaper who became known as one prescribing diets, not pills, misled his audience and viewers of his videos under the guise of being a medical authority. His patients would probably have been better off if he had prescribed them pills for which he had training. As we saw before, nutrition seems simple on its face but in actuality is quite a complex subject and is risky business especially for one who has no training in it.

Dr. Ray Peat, Ph.D., a prominent American physiologist once said, "A few years ago, most of the nutritional problems that I saw were caused by physicians, by refined convenience foods, and by poverty. Recently, most of the problems seem to be caused by badly designed vegetarian diets, or by acceptance of the idea that 40 grams of protein per day is sufficient" [293].

In the vegetarian world, among their gurus are Dean Ornish, M.D., John A. McDougal, M.D., Neal D. Barnard, M.D., Caldwell B. Esselstyn, Jr., M.D., and T. Colin Campbell, Ph.D. One of them, Dr. Barnard the president of the "Physicians Committee for Responsible Medicine," claimed that a low-fat vegan diet can improve diabetes and cardiovas-□ cular risk factors. His two studies, which I discussed in detail previously, showed some improvements in diabetic patients short-term (22 weeks) but when extended to 74 weeks failed to maintain those improvements [278, 279]. In the Spring 2015 issue of the *Good Medicine* magazine, there is a picture with the caption, *The Incredible Inedible Egg*, which is held between two fingers, and there is a label on the egg that reads, "Consuming eggs can significantly increase the risk of diabetes" [294, p.19]. These words sound to me as being incredibly responsible. Right?

Ahrens et al. observed in cases of carbohydrate-induced *lipemia* that "Triglyceride levels were lowest when dietary fat made up 70 percent of the calories and the highest on the high-carbohydrate, low-fat regimen. Figure 4 shows still another feature of this phenomenon: in two patients so tested, when triglycerides were lowest on the high-fat feeding, it made little difference whether the sole dietary fat was corn oil or butter" [286]. As Nina Teicholz showed [133], it appears that butter is good for us, Dr. Klaper. Is it possible that Dr. Klaper based his vegetarian career on faulty premises?

In the above quotes in [286] and in [288, 4:10-6:05], Ahrens and Klaper use the terms "serum" and "plasma" interchangeably. Strictly speaking, there is a difference between them. "Plasma differs from serum in that **serum** is plasma that has been altered in the laboratory to remove fibrinogen (a clotting factor) or some other element that is unwanted in the sample" [62, p.811]. The test tube with Mr. Phillip's blood was not treated in a laboratory, but was just sitting for a few hours, long enough that the blood cells could precipitate and form a jelly-like clot at the lower part of the test tube and plasma would remain above it. Maybe it is not important, but Frayn exclusively uses the term "plasma."

13

PROTEINS

Our bodies can use all three basic macronutrients in food, carbohydrates, fats, and proteins, as sources of energy, while proteins serve as building materials as well. Proteins constitute our muscles, tendons, skin, blood, and organs. They also are an essential component of our bones, hair, teeth, cartilage, and finger-nails. Proteins also play a major role in connective tissue, lymph, hormones, enzymes, blood cells, antibodies, etc.

Proteins are complex molecules, mainly formed of carbon, nitro-gen, and oxygen in various combinations as amino acids (i.e., *amine-*containing nitrogen), which are considered the proteins' building blocks. Our digestive system breaks down proteins into amino acids so that our cells can assimilate them. The most important function of amino acids is to build and maintain muscle mass. Proteins in food provide these needed amino acids for muscle-building.

There are twenty one amino acids needed to maintain health, eight of which humans can not synthesize in adequate amounts from other substances. They are known as *essential amino acids* and they have to be obtained from food. The eight essential amino acids are isoleucine, leucine, lysine, methionine, phenylalanine, threonine, tryptophan, and valine [295]. Two more amino acids, arginine and histidine, are considered essential for children [296].

Essential amino acids are produced by plants during their growth. Nonessential amino acids can be synthesized in our bodies from various substances. Proteins containing sufficient amounts of all eight essential amino acids are present in animal foods, such as meat, poultry, fish, eggs, and dairy products, and plant foods. Beans, peas, lentils, grains, seeds, nuts, vegetables, and fruits are examples of foods lacking or having insufficient quantities of one or more essential amino acids [297].

Vegetarian books and websites on healthy eating claim that all eight essential amino acids can be obtained in adequate quantities from virtually *any* vegetable or whole grain [298]. Indeed, plants such as quinoa, soybeans, peanuts, chia, brown rice, tomatoes, broccoli, and many others contain all essential amino acids and in amounts that people need.

The problem with proteins derived from plants is that plants also contain lectins [12], phytic acid and other anti-nutrients which are less than healthy. Also, plant proteins are incorporated inside plant cells made of cellulose but humans lack cellulase enzymes, required for cellulose metabolism. Ruminant animals possess these enzymes and can process plant foods for us [299]. Ruminants eat plants and we eat ruminants; this is an easy way to obtain a "complete" protein with all essential amino acids without the side effects of plant foods.

Proteins are broken down into amino acids via digestion and reassembled as needed inside our cells. Furthermore, these are needed in adequate quantities. The condition in which the supply and expenditure of amino acids is equal is called "the nitrogen balance." An intake greater than output puts one into "a positive nitrogen balance"; it occurs when the input of amino acids exceeds expenditure [300]. It is worth noting that the best and only food designed by nature to perfectly meet the human baby amino-acid needs is human breast milk.

Although essential amino acids are necessary for various body functions, not all of them are beneficial to our health and longevity. A few studies have shown that two acids– *phenylalanine* and *tyrosine* –

were found to strengthen the immune system and inhibit tumor growth when they were **restricted** in the diet [301].

This applies to a vegetarian diet as well. Plants with a low or moderate content of these amino acids include apples, cabbage, collard greens, mustard greens, and dried figs. High phenylalanine and tyrosine plant-based foods include soybeans, lentils, whole grains, nuts, and seeds. Animal foods with a high content of these two amino acids are cheese, beef, lamb, chicken, pork, fish, eggs, and dairy [302].

Amino acids *tryptophan, methionine* and *cysteine* high in muscle meats are also considered "problem" amino acids. "Although several amino acids can be acutely or chronically toxic, even lethal, when too much is eaten, tryptophan is the only amino acid that is also carcinogenic" [303]. Tryptophan restriction was shown to delay the reproductive age of female rats and slow down the aging process [304].

Methionine restriction "resulted in a 42% increase in mean and 44% increase in maximum life span" in rats [305]. Cysteine and its precursor methionine are the only two sulfur-containing amino acids. In rodents, methionine restricted by 40 %, greatly decreased mitochondrial reactive oxygen species ROS generation and oxidative damage and increased the maximum life span [306].

The methionine content of protein measured in the heart of eight mammalian species ranging in Maximum Life Span (MLS) from 3.5 (mouse) to 46 years (horse) was found to inversely correlate with MLS [307]. To restrict these amino acids "that are associated with many of the problems of aging", Dr. Peat advises to eat gelatin as a major dietary protein. Gelatin contains glycine and proline and "no tryptophan, and only small amounts of cysteine, methionine, and histidine" [308]. Good sources of gelatin is meat stock and bone broth made of oxtail and beef legs.

All three macronutrients, carbohydrates, fat, and protein can be used by our bodies as a source of energy. The efficiency of conversion of these food components into energy is reflected in diet-induced **thermogenesis** (production of heat), an increase of the metabolic rate after a meal. Metabolism of nutrients requires energy that the body provides to break them down, absorb, and assimilate before their energy that is liberated by oxidation becomes available. This is known as *used* energy.

This *used* energy is the lowest, 0 to 3% for fat, higher, 5 to 10% for carbohydrates, and the greatest, 20 to 30% for protein [309]. This means that the lowest cost of fat metabolism makes it the preferred source of energy and protein as the least preferable. Because of that, proteins, which provide the same 4 kcal per gram as carbohydrates, are an ineffective and expensive fuel.

This fact, however, can become beneficial for overweight people and a high-protein diet was proved to be effective for weight loss in a study that lasted for two years [280]. Also, like carbohydrates and fat, protein upon being oxidized for energy creates carbon dioxide CO_2 and water, however proteins leave behind also 'other products.' These 'other products' which are excreted in the urine are: urea 6.065%, ammonia 0.075%, creatinine 0.008%, and sulphuric acid 0.022% [116, p.237].

This means that over 6% of protein is lost to the body as byproducts of metabolism. Therefore, it is important to consume protein in optimal amounts, not too much, otherwise, we can overtax our elimination systems, namely the liver and kidneys.

The presence of all essential amino acids in sufficient amounts defines high-quality protein and many argue that animal proteins are superior than plant proteins [136, p.157]. The plant-based diet advocates contend otherwise [98, p.33]. Both breast milk and eggs, nature's most perfect foods, contain all essential amino acids and in proper proportions. As compared with 1 quart (946 g) of breast milk, one 50g egg contains 63% of leucine and 91% of methionine+cystine. Other amino acids are falling within that range [136, p.77].

Long maligned by official dietary "authorities" because of their high cholesterol content, eggs were eventually exonerated [136, p.88-90]. Dr. Kummerow who dismantled the cholesterol myth and who lived to the age of 102 was a researcher who considered eggs as "the most nutritious and the least expensive protein source in the grocery store [136, p.88]. Commenting on the ad campaign for eggs, "the incredible, edible egg" [310], he wrote, "This certainly is true" [136, p.91].

Myself, I have eaten two eggs a day for years and never worried about their high cholesterol or saturated fat content. I do not bother buying organic eggs, just regular large ones. While I lived in Maine, I happened to visit an organic farm whose owner was a big advocate of sustainable agriculture.

Her chickens were roaming around foraging for worms, bugs and roots while we were waiting for her to come back home. When she returned, she opened a bag with the standard chicken feed from a store (corn and soybeans) and threw handfuls to her chickens. What chickens could pick from the soil was not enough and the bulk of their regimen was still corn and soybeans high in PUFA. For me it was evidence that organic or regular eggs do not differ much.

There are examples of certain persons and scientists experimenting on themselves, who lived for a long period of time on a low-calorie, low-protein, low-fat, and low-carbohydrate intake with emphasis on real and wholesome foods. Some of the diets, such as Dr. Galina Shatalova's diet with its mere 20 g/day of protein, 100 g/day of carbohydrates and 700 to 1,000 kcal/day intake, may seem to be an extreme, semi-starvation diet.

However, Dr. Shatalova (1916–2011), MD, Ph.D., the Russian neurosurgeon who had two heart attacks at the age of 59, applied it to herself, became healthy again and lived to the age of 95. As a scientist and physician involved in the Russian astronauts' nutrition research, she enjoyed her own good health and helped thousands of her patients [311].

A 113-year-old Singaporean, Teresa Hsu (1898-2011), also lived on very little food. Her breakfast usually consisted of a glass of water (0 kcal) or milk (150 kcal). She often had milk (150 kcal) and salad for lunch, or food that people sometimes brought her (probably 300 to 400 kcal). Dinner was milk or yogurt (150 kcal) [312]. The daily total was about 800 kcal. "You waste energy digesting unnecessary food!" she was reported as saying in the November 7, 1997, issue of *The Straits Times,* a Singapore newspaper.

Although a raw food diet is all the rage, no long living culture has lived on all raw food. A raw food diet means that all the foods a person eats are raw, uncooked plant foods. It is considered an extreme diet and people who engage in eating only raw foods are regarded as experimenting on themselves.

Almost every nutritionist, physician and even some ex-raw food enthusiasts [313] will tell you about numerous dangers, including bacteria and germs; indigestion; a deficiency of essential amino acids, minerals, and vitamins D and B12; the hazards of surviving on low-calorie raw food in winter, and many others. I tried a raw food diet for one year and a half and found that it did not work for me.

The people who have lived on a raw-food diet for years and even decades will tell you instead that eating cooked food is the fastest way to acquire many degenerative diseases, age rapidly, and die prematurely. The most powerful argument in favor of eating raw foods is the preservation of digestive enzymes in food, which otherwise are easily destroyed in cooking [314]. The raw food diet was discussed in more detail in my previous book [259].

14

HOW MUCH PROTEIN DO WE NEED?

T he other question is about the amount of protein we need. Many physicians and nutritionists believe that too much protein is harmful. Excessive protein intake for a prolonged period is linked to serious degenerative illnesses such as heart disease, cancer, stroke, kidney failure, diabetes, and many others [315].

On the other hand, too little protein consumption leads to malnutrition, a condition also dangerous to our health. The healthy amount, if established, cannot be a fixed amount, because it is very dependent on a person's body constitution, blood type, lifestyle, and activities, as well as climate, season, environmental conditions and other factors.

The scientific estimation of protein requirements for a human body is based on measurements of nitrogen losses (i.e., in urine, feces, skin shedding, and perspiration) in experimental subjects who were put on a protein-free diet [316]. Our total daily nitrogen losses must be replenished with nitrogen derived from dietary protein. The protein requirement for body maintenance is determined to be an average of 0.34 gram of protein per kilogram (2.2 pounds) of body weight per day, or 25 grams for a 160-pound (73-kilogram) man. The U.S. RDA is 0.8 gram of protein per kilogram (2.2 pounds) of body weight per day, or

58 grams for a male of the same body weight, or 60 grams of protein in a 2,000-kcal diet [317].

Natural-health advocates are much stricter when it comes to protein consumption. Their sole concern is the amount of dietary protein necessary for the replacement of body protein, which is lost daily by dead cells broken down during metabolic processes. Protein is not considered being an energy source.

According to Dr. Galina Shatalova of Moscow, Russia, who lived to age 95, the daily protein intake necessary to maintain the body weight of an adult human is estimated to be 0.25 gram per kilogram of body mass [311]. For an adult with a body weight of 160 pounds (73 kilograms), this means 18.3 grams of protein a day.

A somewhat higher figure is stated in the book *Fit for Life* by Harvey and Marilyn Diamond, who say that to maintain weight, the human body needs to replenish a daily loss of 23 grams of protein, which is very close to the previously mentioned scientific estimate. Protein is lost in feces and urine, from growing hair and nails, sloughed-off skin, and perspiration. Following H. & M. Diamond, the human body recycles 70 percent of the protein waste within the body before the remainder is eliminated from the body mainly in the feces and urine [318, p.88].

The recycling of amino acids is key to understanding why we need so little protein. Back in 1957, Rose, W.C. estimated that 18 grams of protein a day would be sufficient for adult men to provide all amino acids [319]. In 1963, Hegsted suggested that we need a mere 10 grams of protein a day, considering that our body is very efficient in recycling amino acids [320].

An amount close to this figure is stated in *The Optimum Nutrition Bible*, by Patrick Holford, one of Britain's leading nutritional authors and the founder of the Institute for Optimum Nutrition in London. He states, "At the low end of the scale are reports of protein sufficiency when 2.5 percent of total calorie intake comes from protein" [4, p.34]. For a 2,000-kcal diet, it recommends 50 kcal or 12.5 grams of protein.

Actually, it is very difficult to design a 2,000-kcal diet with such a tiny amount of protein because protein is in everything. A person must eat only low-protein plants such as apples and cucumbers. For instance, twenty apples (80 kcal each) and six cucumbers (40 kcal each), which comprise 12.5 grams of protein, would total only 1,840 kcal.

For therapeutic purposes, amounts as low as 0.2 gram per kilogram of body weight reportedly have been used with significant effects in the treatment of patients with kidney failure for a prolonged period. For a 160 pound (73-kilogram) male, this translates into 14.6 grams of protein per day [321].

Although animal protein is a kind of test for our digestive system, we need it. Biologically, we are less suited for all meat-eating as are carnivorous animals. They have a short intestine, very strong digestive juices (ten times stronger than ours), and the meat they eat passes in 3 to 4 hours. Our intestine is three times longer, our digestive juices are weak (especially in Blood type A1 people), and for most people, it takes 24 to 48 hours for meat to pass. The acid environment favorable for the breakdown of meat exists only in the stomach, where meat stays only a few hours. Therefore, little meat (i.e., about 3 ounces for blood type A1 and 4 ounces for blood type O) can be properly digested at one time; larger amounts pass through the intestines only partly digested.

However, meat provides all necessary amino acids in higher concentrations than other protein sources, as the study published in 2016 shows. "Intakes of all 18 dietary amino acids differed by diet group; for the majority of these, intake was highest in meat-eaters followed by fish-eaters, then vegetarians and lowest in vegans (up to 47% lower than in meat-eaters)" [322].

Animal protein, like our muscle protein, has a very complex structure and a significant amount of energy is necessary to break it down to molecules that can be utilized by the cells. A small part of protein is used to replace dead cells, for maintenance and repair; the significant part is converted to glucose through the process of gluconeogenesis and then burned for energy. It is commonly known that meat is a heavy food for digestion. It is quite an energy-consuming process and our body must first expend calories in order to later get these calories back through the metabolism of the meat. In a high-protein, carbohydrate-free diet, the protein metabolism energy expenditure is as high as 42% [323].

Digesting meat is like an internal workout and our body must sweat a lot to do the job. This is probably one of the reasons why people on a high-protein diet lose weight–they do not need to go to the gym because they have one inside. Their bodies are already engaged in strenuous exercise digesting the meat.

For some people, vegetable protein can serve as an alternative to animal protein apparently without adverse effects. Discussing a healthy amount of vegetable protein intake, Drs. Agatha and Calvin Thrash, in their book *Nutrition for Vegetarians,* assert that amounts of 25 to 40 grams from vegetable foods could be sufficient [324]. Living proof that an individual can survive taking the lowest level in that range was Dr. Norman Walker (1886-1985), who daily consumed 25 grams of protein by eating exclusively raw fruits and vegetables, nuts, and some cheese; he lived to 99 years and five months [325].

In some cultures, low meat consumption was a part of the lifestyle for centuries. Consider the Japanese, who traditionally eat little meat, mostly fish, rice, and sea and land vegetables. They are slim and rarely have heart disease. Their polar opposites are sumo wrestlers (by their profession) are models of obesity.

For centuries, their diet was based on rice and vegetables; however, in the last sixty years, meat has been added. They have become heavier and heavier with every passing decade. A wrestler's average weight of 317 pounds in 1953 is now 412 pounds, and their life span is sixteen years shorter than that of the average Japanese male. "The incidence of diabetes mellitus, gout, and hypertension in wrestlers was 5.2, 6.3, and 8.3%, respectively, all values being considerably higher than in controls" [326].

The same happened to Japanese from Okinawa who emigrated to Brazil at the beginning of the twentieth century. They relocated with their great longevity genes, but adopted a local lifestyle with abundant meat (as much as 2 pounds a day) in the diet. As a result, 25 percent of the transplanted Japanese suffered from diabetes and lived fifteen to seventeen years less than their peers in Japan [327].

These examples reveal that overconsumption of calories in sumo wrestlers and meat in Brazilian Okinawans entails adverse health consequences. However, a study of the Japanese elderly showed health and longevity benefits from moderately increased content of animal protein in their diets. "Nutrient intakes in 94 Japanese centenarians investigated between 1972 and 1973 showed a higher proportion of animal protein to total proteins than in contemporary average Japanese" [328].

15

EXCESSIVE PROTEIN CONSUMPTION
AND CANCER

A diet containing too much protein, especially animal protein, can lead to cancer, says Dr. A. Vogel in his widely acclaimed book, *Swiss Nature Doctor*. Excessive protein intake leads to constant irritation of the cells, thus encouraging abnormal cell growth, adds Dr.Vogel [329, p. 225]. The publication *Diet, Nutrition, and Cancer* of the National Academy of Sciences suggests that high protein intake may increase the risk of cancer of the breast, colon, rectum, pancreas, prostate gland, and kidneys [330]. Michio Kushi, in his book *The Cancer Prevention Diet,* ascribes animal protein to be the primary high-risk factor in the development of many types of cancer [331]. The countries with a high protein consumption have higher death rates from cancer, as shown in Figure 15-4.

Although the scatter in Figure 15-4 is quite large, the correlation between protein consumption and the death rate is quite distinctive. A highest death rate is found in Hungary; Denmark, with its protein consumption of approximately 100 grams per day, is second. Other European countries with high protein consumption, including the United Kingdom, Belgium, France, Italy, and Germany, are shown in the upper right portion of the graph.

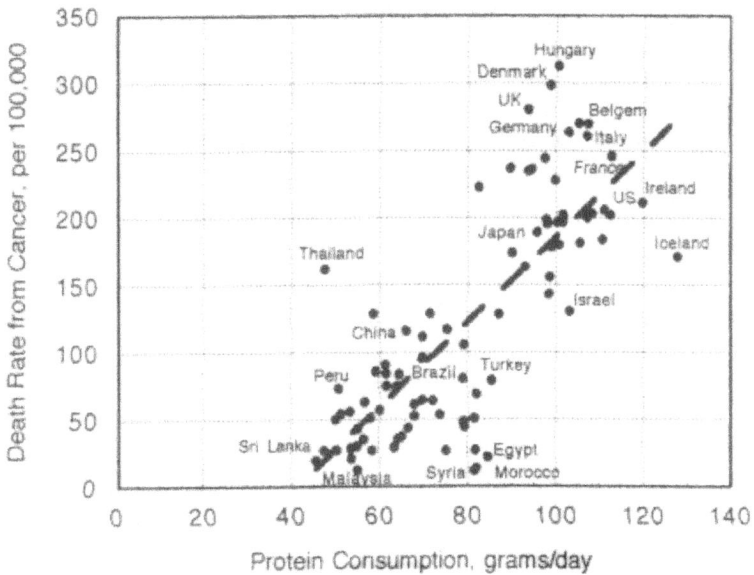

Figure 15-4. Death Rate from Cancer vs. Protein Consumption in 87 Countries

Although protein consumption is among the highest in the United States, Ireland, and France, the death rate from cancer is close to the averanging line. Iceland with its highest (127.9 grams per day) protein consumption, enjoys a lower than average death rate.

Among the countries with low protein consumption, Thailand is way above the line because of air pollution in Bangkok, men over smoking, and extremely spicy foods that irritate the digestive tract and which contribute to the development of lung and colon cancers [332]. China is close to the line and Malaysia is below it. The Arab countries including Egypt, Syria and Morocco enjoy the lowest death rate despite a medium protein consumption of about 80 grams per day [333], perhaps because of fasting during Ramadan.

In this discussion, I am not trying to claim that excessive protein causes cancer; rather, combined with other risk factors, it may promote the development of cancer. Research studies show that ill-absorbed protein, such as derived from processed meats, when entering the colon, may disrupt beneficial bacteria and, in extreme cases, can cause colon cancer [334].

Because excessive intake of protein may be detrimental to a person's health, the global question is whether food is the only source of protein for our bodies, or are there other sources? This matter is discussed in chapter 16 of my book, "Control for Life ...." [259].

16

CONCLUSION

T he review and analysis of nutrition and diets conducted herein allow us to arrive at the following conclusions:

1. Fats became and still remain the most misunderstood part of our nutrition. As opposed to "official" health advice, saturated fats are stable and not subject to oxidative damage. Coconut oil, butter and beef fat (tallow) with their highest saturated fat content are the healthiest of all fats. Polyunsaturated fatty acids PUFAs in vegetable oils undergo many stages of oxidative damage in the process of extraction, refining, deodorization and using them for deep frying, create toxic aldehydes, and therefore are most deleterious to health.

2. *Trans* fats that are created in vegetable oils in the process of hydrogenation as well as during deodorization, refining, and deep frying are linked to many serious health problems such as heart disease, stroke, cancer, and diabetes. *Trans* fats are universally accepted as toxic and banned in the United States. Although food producers claim 0% of *trans* fats on food labels, if analyzed, they can be found in foods deep-fried in vegetable oils.

3. Polyunsaturated fats are subject to oxidation and formation of toxic aldehydes and hence can have the opposite effect in health and disease. Omega 3 and omega 6 fatty acids can make a healthy person

sick and even initiate and promote cancer in them but can kill cancer cells in a person so stricken.

4. The issue of healthy fats is very important for the overall health of Blood type A1 people, which comprise 33.6% of the US population. Their average life expectancy is the shortest, only 62 years, as compared to the 87 years of blood type Os. A1s are the most vulner□ able of all Blood types. Heart disease, stroke, cancer, and diabetes kill Blood type A1 people prematurely. The proposed Blood type A1 diet can help such people become healthier and live longer.

5. The current policy of avoiding animal fat and lowering blood cholesterol for prevention and treatment of cardiovascular disease has a serious drawback: an increased risk of cancer death.

6. Carbohydrates can have deleterious effects to our health. They trigger the secretion of hormones (growth factors) such as insulin and insulin-like growth factors IGF 1 and IGF 2, which can lead to cancer growth. The advanced glycation end products (AGEs) in which protein molecules are stiffened and degraded in an irreversible way are formed while cooking at high temperatures.

Carbohydrates taken in excess can cause a disorder called *lipemia*, or "fatty blood." The concentration of triglycerides in the blood is increased through the process of *de novo* lipogenesis in which the liver creates fats from glucose. The proponents of the low fat, plant-based diet erroneously accuse animal fat and cholesterol of causing *lipemia* and thus base their movement's philosophy on false premises.

7. Proteins are broken down into amino acids by our digestive system so that the body can assimilate them. Among *essential amino acids*, tryptophan, methionine, and cysteine that are high in muscle meats are considered "problem" amino acids. Tryptophan was found to be carcinogenic and restriction of these three amino acids has resulted in an increased life span in rodents. As compared to muscle meats, gelatin contains only small amounts of cysteine, methionine, and histidine and can serve as a main source of protein. A good source of gelatin is meat stock and bone broth made from oxtails and beef legs.

8. The protein amount in the proposed Blood type A1 diet is optimal. For a 5'11" (180 cm) individual, the protein requirements would

be 64 grams (2.25 oz). Excessive protein consumption (over 100g/day) is associated with different kinds of cancer and rich nations with high protein consumption have higher death rates from cancer. Temperance and moderation, the motto of long-lived people and cente-☐ narians, once again holds sway.

Appendix 1

In this Blood Type A1 diet, first in the morning:

A cup of herbal or green tea with 1 Tbsp coconut oil, 1 tsp raw honey, and 1 Tbsp Apple cider vinegar.

BREAKFAST
Energy smoothie.
Ingredients:

1. Carrot, 1 medium
2. Aloe vera, 1 oz
3. Seaweed, 2 oz
4. Pineapple, 3 oz
5. Coconut meat, 1 oz
6. Cilantro, 0.2 oz
7. Raisins, 1 Tbsp
8. Asparagus, 1 oz
9. Ginger, 1 oz
10. Plantain, raw, 3 oz
11. Habanero pepper, 1/3 tsp (tincture preparation)
12. Garlic, 0.2 oz
13. Orange juice, 1 cup
14. Sea salt, 1 tsp (6g)
15. Okra, frozen, 1 oz
16. Pomegranate, 0.5 oz
17. Purified water,1 cup

I blend it for 2 minutes in the Vita Mix blender.

LUNCH
Alternating carrots 3.5 oz, cucumber, lettuce, blueberries
I cup of bone broth/meat stock
or pumpkin (2 oz) and rice (1 oz) soup with I cup of bone broth/meat stock as a base
Coconut oil, 2 Tbsp
Jams, apricot, 20g
Mushrooms, 1 oz

DINNER

Appetizer 1
1. Grated carrots, 3 oz
2. Grated beets, 2 oz
3. Palm oil, 1 Tbsp (14 g)
4. Vinegar, 1 Tbsp
5. Fruit preserve, 1 Tbsp
Appetizer 2
1. Butter, 1.5 oz
2. Caviar, 1/4 tsp

Main dish:

1. Two scrambled eggs cooked with 1 Tbsp coconut oil, sea salt, black pepper to taste

or 1 can (4 oz) of crab meat, 2 scrambled eggs (44g medium size) cooked with 1 Tbsp coconut oil, sea salt, black pepper to taste, and salmon, 2 oz,

or 1 can of oysters, 2 scrambled eggs cooked with 1 Tbsp coconut oil, sea salt, black pepper to taste

or 3.2 oz beef/lamb, ground, fatty, not lean, with 2 scrambled eggs cooked with 1 Tbsp coconut oil, sea salt, black pepper to taste.

2. Green onions, 1 oz.
3. Onions, 1 oz.
4. Romaine lettuce, 1 oz.
5. Olives, 2 oz
6. Sauerkraut, 1 Tbsp
7. Kim chi, 1 oz
8. Honey, 1 Tbsp
9. Red grape wine, 4 fl. oz

Sip wine in the course of the meal.† Dinner is eaten 3 hours before bed. To ensure proper digestion of the animal proteins, no liquids are taken after dinner.

----

† People with liver disease such as hepatitis should avoid drinking any alcoholic beverages including wine.

SHOPPING LIST

All real, whole, natural foods, no processed, man-made foods.
Preferably all foods are organic.

***Warning: Different blood types can have allergic reactions to
various foods in the following list. Please check with Table 9 of
the Dr. Laura Power study for your specific blood type [25].***

1. butter
2. caviar
3. coconut oil
4. macadamia nut oil

5. beef, cow's liver, tail, heart, kidneys, internal fat, bones with marrow, tongue, bone broth, stock

6. lamb, it's liver, tail, heart, kidneys, internal fat, bones with marrow, tongue, bone broth, stock

7. asparagus*
8. beets*
9. carrots*
10. celery*
11. cucumber*
12. lettuce salad*
13. pumpkin, squash*
14. cayenne pepper**
15. Ceylon cinnamon**
16. garlic**
17. ginger**
18. onions**
19. pineapple**
20. pomegranate**
21. turmeric, curry**
22. aloe vera
23. apple cider vinegar
24. bananas
25. black pepper
26. blueberries
27. chives
28. chocolate
29. cilantro
30. cinnamon
31. clams
32. coconut, coconut flour, coconut milk, and cream
33. cod
34. coffee
35. crab meat, canned
36. cranberries
37. dates
38. dandelion greens
39. dill
40. eggs
41. figs
42. fruit preserves
43. honey, raw, unfiltered
44. lemons and lemon juice
45. limes and lime juice
46. lobster
47. olives
48. oranges and orange juice
49. oysters, canned
50. parsley
51. plantains

52. plums
53. prunes
54. raisins
55. sardines in brine or hot sauce
56. scallions
57. seaweed (except kombu or nori)
58. sea salt
59. tea green, herbal
60. water, reverse osmosis, refilled in glass bottles
61. watermelon

----

* Negative calorie foods   ** Blood thinners

NUTRITIONAL VALUE

This diet provides (% of Daily Value DV):

Calories: 2270
Protein: 71.9 g (13%)
Carbohydrates: 137 g (23%)
Glycemic Load: 53 of 100
Fiber: 18.6 g
Starch: 1.4 g
Sugar: 86.1 g
Fat: 158 g (60%)
Saturated fat: 112 g
Monounsaturated fat: 28.4 g
Polyunsaturated fat: 5.7 g
omega 3, ω-3: 1.057 g
omega 6, ω-6: 4.537 g
Cholesterol: 272 mg (91%)
Phytosterols: 105 mg
Trans fats: 0.0 g
Alcohol: 13.7 g (4%)
Water: 1181g
Ash: 18.6 g

AMINO ACIDS:
Tryptophan: 657 mg
Methionine: 1396 mg
Cystine: 758 mg
VITAMINS:
Vit. A: 25089 IU (502 %)
Vit. C: 241 mg (402 %)
Vit. D: 68 IU (17 %)
Vit. E: 5.9 mg (30 %)
Vit. K: 224 mcg (280 %)
Thiamin: 0.9 mg (57 %)
Riboflavin: 1.7 mg (97 %)
Niacin: 18.2 mg (91 %)
Vit. B6: 1.5 mg (77 %)
Folate: 377 mcg (94 %)
Vit. B12: 7.4 mcg (124 %)
Pantothenic acid: 5.0 mg (50 %)
Choline: 164 mg
Betaine: 6.9 mg

MINERALS:

Ca: 594 mg (59% DV), Mg: 233 mg (58% DV), P: 883 mg (88% DV), K: 3728 mg (155% DV), Na: 3038 mg (87% DV), I: 11.1 mg (62% DV), Zn: 98 mg (66% DV), Co: 1.5 mg (78% DV), Mn: 3.0 mg (150% DV), Se: 65.6 mcg (94% DV).

GLOSSARY

aging — the decline of any physiological, cellular or biochemical functions that occurs over time rather than from injury or disease and accompanied by a diminished probability of survival.

aldehydes — oxidation products created in the breakdown of peroxidized fats having cross-linking, mutagenic and carcinogenic properties.

Alzheimer's disease — a chronic, progressive, degenerative cognitive disorder beginning with memory loss and progressing to deterioration of intellectual functions, personality changes, and speech and language problems.

amino acids — building blocks of proteins and the end products of protein digestion.

ammonia — an alkaline gas formed by decomposition of nitrogen containing substances such as proteins and amino acids. In the body, all blood gases including ammonia are in solution.

anti-nutrients — natural and synthetic compounds in plant foods such as digestive enzyme (protease and amylase) inhibitors, phytic acid, and lectins (hemagglutinins) that inhibit the absorption of nutrients, e.g. iron and calcium, and can cause mineral and niacin deficiencies.

apoptosis — programmed death of cells, may limit growth of tumors.

arteriosclerosis — a disease of the arterial blood vessels marked by thickening, hardening and loss of elasticity in the arterial walls.

arthritis — joint inflammation, often accompanied by pain, swelling, stiffness, and deformity.

atherosclerosis — the most common form of arteriosclerosis, marked by oxidized cholesterol-lipid-calcium deposits in the walls of arteries that may restrict blood flow and cause heart attack or stroke.

Ayurveda — an ancient Indian Traditional Medicine which takes into account body constitution determined by three metabolic principles or doshas: Vata, Pitta and Kapha. It incorporates exercise, balanced diet, detoxification, herbs, and various techniques to stimulate the circulation of prana or life force.

bile — a viscous fluid secreted by the liver which emulsifies fats facilitating their digestion in the small intestines by pancreatic lipase.

biochemistry — the science of the chemical changes accompanying the vital functions of plants and animals.

Blood groups or types — a genetically determined system of antigens located on the surface of red blood cells. The ABO system is of a prime importance in blood transfusions. The most common are the four blood groups: O, A, B and AB.

"blue zones" — the geographical regions of exceptional longevity.

body constitution — the physical makeup and functional habits of the body.

butyric acid — a short-chain saturated fatty acid C4:0, a component of bovine milk and also derived from bacterial fermentation of dietary fiber in the bowel.

cardiovascular disease — any disease of the heart or blood vessels, including atherosclerosis, disease affecting heart muscles (cardiomyopathy), coronary artery disease, peripheral vascular disease, and others.

centenarian — a person over the age of 100.

cholesterol — a sterol synthesized in the liver and a normal constituent of bile serving as a precursor of various steroid hormones such as sex hormones, adrenal corticoids, Vitamin D and widely distributed in body tissues. Dietary cholesterol comes from egg yolks, animal fat and organ meats, e.g. liver and kidneys.

Cochrane Collaboration — an international group of academics that performs systematic reviews of published health care research and study the effectiveness of medical treatments.

C-reactive protein — an indicator of inflammation in arteries, a predictor of heart attack risk.

creatinine — the decomposition product of the phospho-creatine metabolism, a source of energy for muscle contraction.

Crohn's disease — an inflammatory bowel disease marked by patchy areas of full-thickness inflammation in the gastrointestinal tract.

dementia — a progressive, irreversible decline in mental function, marked by memory impairment, and, often, deficits of reasoning, judgement, abstract thought, comprehension, learning, task performance, and use of language.

de novo **lipogenesis** — formation of fat in the liver from other substrates, e.g. glucose, fatty acids or amino acids.

diabetes — a chronic metabolic disorder marked by elevated blood glucose levels (hyperglycemia) and excessive urination. It results either from failure of the pancreas to produce insulin (type 1 diabetes) or from insulin resistance, with inadequate insulin secretion to sustain normal metabolism (type 2 diabetes).

diarrhea — the passage of fluid or unformed stools.

edema (fluid retention) — a condition in which body tissues contain an excessive amount of tissue fluid.

ejaculation — ejection of the seminal fluid from the male urethra, male orgasm.

endothelial injury — damage to the endothelial cells that line artery wall caused by oxidized cholesterol, lipid peroxidation aldehydes, e.g. MDA, HNE and HHE, smoking, diabetes, high blood pressure, elevated C-reactive protein and homocysteine, and others.

enzymes — proteins that catalyze biochemical reactions without changing their own structure.

epigenetics — changes in gene expression due to lifestyle factors such as diet and behavioral habits, and the environment.

estrogen — the female sex hormone secreted by the ovary (gland producing reproductive cells).

eunuch — a castrated man.

fasting — going without food or other nutritional support.

fecal transplantation — the transfer of stool from a healthy donor into the gastrointestinal tract for the purpose of treating recurrent C. difficile colitis or other gut conditions.

Framingham Heart Study — a study of the risk factors that contribute to the development of coronary artery disease and stroke performed with a group of about 5000 residents of Framingham, MA.

free radicals — highly reactive molecules containing an odd number of electrons, having an open bond and creating oxidative stress.

French paradox — the unexpectedly low rate of heart disease in France despite a typically high-fat diet.

gelatin — a protein obtained by the hydrolysis of collagen present in the connective tissues of the skin, bones, and joints of animals.

ghee — a form of clarified butter made from cow's milk and traditionally used in Asian cooking.

growth hormone — a hormone secreted by the anterior pituitary gland and regulating the cell division and protein synthesis necessary for normal growth.

hepatitis — acute or chronic inflammation of the liver, usually caused by exposure to an infectious agent (e.g., a hepatitis virus), a toxin (e.g., alcohol), or a drug (e.g., acetaminophen).

HHE, 4-hydroxy-2-nonenal — reactive and cytotoxic product of peroxidation of the PUFA containing oils and fats. It was detected in inflammatory situations such as atherosclerotic lesions, in the brain of Alzheimer's and other neurophysiological disease patients.

HNE, 4-hydroxy-2-hexanal — highly reactive and toxic product of peroxidation of omega-6 containing fats and oils. HNE has been linked to such diseases as cataracts, Alzheimer's, atherosclerosis, diabetes, and cancer.

homocysteine — an amino acid which is an intermediate product in the metabolism of methionine and cysteine.

insulin-like growth factor (IGF) — a hormone that functions as the major mediator of growth hormone GH -stimulated growth of cells. For example, IGF-1 that is synthesized in the liver and secreted into the blood is under the control of GH.

interleukin — any of a class of glycoproteins (proteins that have carbohydrate groups attached to the polypeptide chain) produced by leukocytes (white blood cells) for regulating immune responses.

ketogenic diet — low carbohydrates, high fat (over 80%) diet particularly suitable for weight loss.

ketones — substances, e.g. acetone, derived from fatty acids as a source of fuel when glucose is at a short supply or there is not enough insulin in the blood.

lactic acid — substrate (substance acted upon) of glucose breakdown or synthesis (gluconeogenesis) in the liver, muscles and other tissues.

lauric acid — medium-chain saturated fatty acid C12:0 which has a variety of health benefits, including antibacterial, antiviral, antifungal and anticancer properties.

lectins — plant proteins that bind specifically to certain sugars, cause agglutination of particular cell types and stimulate lymphocytes to proliferate.

lipid peroxidation — a process under which free radicals attack and damage lipids (fats) containing double bonds, especially polyunsaturated fatty acids PUFAs.

Longevity Quotient LQ — the ratio of actual observed longevity of a specie to that predicted by their body size.

lysine — a basic amino acid which is a constituent of most proteins and is an essential nutrient in the diet.

malondialdehyde MDA — a byproduct of lipid (fat) metabolism in the body, a marker of lipid peroxidation. It is also found in many foods, especially those fried in vegetable oils, and can be present in high amounts in rancid food.

macular degeneration — an eye disease that progressively destroys the macula, the very center of the retina, impairing central vision.

Mediterranean diet — a presumed traditional in Mediterranean countries diet, characterized especially by a high consumption of vegetables and olive oil and moderate consumption of protein, and thought to confer health benefits.

medium-chain triglycerides MCTs — made by processing coconut and palm kernel oils in the laboratory (partially man-made fats).

metabolism — the chemical processes that occur within a living organism in order to maintain life.

metabolic syndrome — a cluster of biochemical and physiological abnormalities associated with the development of cardiovascular disease and type 2 diabetes.

metabolic waste — substances left over from metabolic processes (such as cellular respiration) which cannot be used by the organism (they are surplus or toxic), and must therefore be excreted. This includes nitrogen compounds, carbon dioxide, phosphates, sulphates, etc.

methionine— a sulfur-containing essential (must be obtained from diet) amino acid that is a constituent of most proteins.

myocardial infarction MI — another term for heart attack.

naked mole rats — nearly blind and hairless mice-like creatures living in large underground colonies in eastern Africa and marked by exceptional longevity.

nitrogen balance — nitrogen intake minus nitrogen loss. Sources of nitrogen intake include meat, dairy, eggs, nuts and legumes, and grains and cereals. Examples of nitrogen losses are urine, feces, sweat, hair, and skin shedding.

obesity — the metabolic/nutritional disease marked by the unhealthy accumulation of body fat and defined as having a body mass index BMI of greater than 30 kg/m.^{2}

oxidation — a process of a substance combining with oxygen acting as a free radical and damaging it by stealing electrons.

oxytocin — a hormone secreted by the hypothalamus and stored in the pituitary gland. It causes the uterus to contract; in breastfeeding and it stimulates milk letdown.

palmitic acid — a solid long-chain saturated fatty acid C16:0 obtained from palm oil and other vegetable and animal fats.

peroxidability index PI — a measure of susceptibility of fatty acids to oxidation; its value increases as the number of double bonds is increased.

phytic acid — an anti-nutrient in grains which impairs the absorption of iron, zinc and calcium and may cause mineral deficiencies.

Progesterone — a steroid hormone released by the **corpus luteum** that stimulates the uterus to prepare for pregnancy.

Prolactin — a hormone released from the anterior pituitary gland that stimulates milk production after childbirth.

purines — a compound found in alcoholic beverages, fish, seafood and meats, especially organ meats like liver. Upon oxidation, it forms uric acid.

reactive carbonyl compounds — highly reactive molecules often known for their damaging effects on proteins, nucleic acids, and lipids.

reactive oxygen species ROS— free radicals that contain oxygen and easily can react with other molecules in a cell causing damage to the cell's DNA, RNA, proteins, and can even cause cell death.

rheumatoid arthritis — a chronic inflammatory disorder that can affect joints and other body parts.

ruminants — polygastric (many stomachs) animals such as cattle, sheep, antelopes, deer, giraffes, and their relatives that chew the cud regurgitated from their rumen.

semen — the male reproductive fluid, containing spermatozoa in suspension.

stearic acid — a common natural waxy solid, the saturated fatty acid C 18:0 occurring as the glyceride in tallow and other animal fats and in some animal oils; used chiefly in the manufacture of soaps, candles, and cosmetics,

stroke — a disease that affects the arteries leading to and within the brain. It occurs when a blood vessel that carries oxygen and nutrients to the brain is either blocked by a clot or bursts (ruptures).

sumo wrestlers — Japanese heavyweight wrestlers; a contestant wins a bout by forcing his opponent outside a marked circle or by making him touch the ground with any part of his body except the soles of his feet.

testosterone — a male sex hormone that is responsible for maturation of the male sexual organs, development of sperm within the testes, sexual drive, and erections of the penis.

thiobarbituric acid TBA — a reagent to detect the thiobarbituric acid reactive substances TBARS which are formed as a byproduct of lipid peroxidation.

thyroid gland — a large ductless gland in the neck which secretes hormones regulating growth and development governs the rate of metabolism.

toxins, endogenous — toxins produced by the body as a byproduct of biochemical processes, and may accumulate in the joints or various muscle groups.

toxins, exogenous — toxins acquired by the body through ingestion, breathing, skin contact or sometimes by injection or other medical treatment.

Traditional Chinese Medicine — a traditional medical system of Chinese origin based on more than 2,500 years of practice that includes various forms of herbal medicine, acupuncture, massage, exercise (qigong), and dietary therapy.

urea — a final product of protein metabolism in the body along with carbon dioxide; it represents a bulk of urinary nitrogen and is increased with a high protein diet.

uric acid — an end product of purine metabolism. It is a common constituent of urinary stones and gouty crystals.

vitality — exuberant physical strength or mental vigor.

weight loss — a measurable decline in body weight, either intentionally or as a result of malnutrition or illness.

World Health Organization WHO — the United Nations agency concerned with international health and the eradication of disease.

worry — to experience anxiety or serious unease; allow one's mind to excessively dwell on difficulties or troubles.

yoga — a system of traditional Hindu beliefs, rituals, and activities that aims to provide spiritual enlightenment and self-knowledge. In the Western world, the term has been associated primarily with physical postures (asanas) and coordinated, diaphragmatic breathing (pranayama).

zinc — a common element essential for proper bodily function and development which is involved in most metabolic processes. Its deficiency is linked to retarded growth and dwarfism, and altered wound healing.

References

1. Wells, Herbert G., Huxley, Julian S. and Wells, G.P. The Science of Life. Garden City, N.Y.: Doubleday, Doran & Company, Inc., 1931. https://www.biblio.com/the-science-of-life-by-wells-h-g/work/170795 (Accessed 04/17/2019)

2. Bieler, H. Food Is Your Best Medicine. Ballantine Books, New York, 1982.

3. Yamamoto S. and McCarty P. Whole Health Shiatsu. Tokyo and New York: Japan Publications, Inc., 1993.

4. Holford, P. The Optimum Nutrition Bible. Freedom, CA: The Crossing Press, 1999.

5. Wallach, JD & Lan, M. Dead Doctors Don't Lie. Legacy communications Group, Franklin Tennessee, 1999.

6. Cooper LF, Barber EM and Mitchell H S. Nutrition in Health and Disease, 7th ed. J. B. Lippincott Company, 1938.

7. http://www.loveandtruth.net/shelton-fasting.html (Accessed 05/17/2019)

8. https://answers.yahoo.com/question/index?qid=20080213133158AAAIvEw (Accessed 05/17/ 2019)

9. https://www.britannica.com/science/extrasensory-perception (Accessed 05/17/ 2019)

10. Roland, P. New Age Living: A Guide to Principles, Practices and Beliefs. Octopus Publishing Group, Ltd., London, 2000.

11. D'Adamo, P. with Whitney, C. Eat Right 4 your Type: The Individualized Diet Solution to Staying Healthy, Living Longer & Achieving Your Ideal Weight. Putnam's Sons, New York, 1996.

12. Gundry, SR. with Buehl, OB. The plant paradox: the hidden dangers in "healthy" foods that cause disease and weight gain. Harper Collins Publishers, New York, 2017.

13. Li, H. et al. Evaluating and predicting the oxidative stability of vegetable oils with different fatty acid compositions. J Food Sci._ 2013

Apr;78(4):H633-41. doi: 10.1111/1750-3841.12089. Epub 2013 Mar 25. (Accessed 05/17/ 2019)

14. Pearce, ML and Dayton, S. Incidence of Cancer in Men on a Diet High in Polyunsaturated Fat. Lancet 297 (7697), 1971, 464-7.

15. https://kresserinstitute.com/goitrogenic-foods-and-thyroid-health/ (Accessed 05/17/ 2019)

16. http://haydeninstitute.com/diet-nutrition-blog/ inflammatory-foods-nightshades (Accessed 05/17/ 2019)

17. https://blog.paleohacks.com/top-11-goitrogenic-foods-thyroid-health/ (Accessed 05/17/ 2019)

18. https://www.healthline.com/nutrition/benefits-of-sauerkraut (Accessed 05/17/ 2019)

19. Daniel, KT. The Whole Soy Story: The Dark side of the America's Favorite Health Food. News Trends, 2004.

20. https://www.sciencedirect.com/topics/agricultural-and-biological-sciences/monogastric (Accessed 05/17/ 2019)

21. http://nutritiondata.self.com/facts/cereal-grains-and-pasta/5687/2 (Accessed 05/17/ 2019)

22. http://nutritiondata.self.com/facts/legumes-and-legume-products/ 4382/2 (Accessed 05/17/ 2019)

23. Bauman, D. E., J. W. Perfield II, M. J. de Veth, and A. L. Lock. New perspectives on lipid digestion and metabolism in ruminants. Proc. Cornell Nutr. Conf. 2003; 175-189.
https://pdfs.semanticscholar.org/bf6a/ d4956581c03ff5df9dc6b2e88fc082f382ad.pdf (Accessed 05/17/ 2019)

24. Hayes DP. Nutritional hormesis. Eur J Clin Nutr. 2007 Feb;61(2): 147-59.

25. https://patents.google.com/patent/US7601509B2/en (Accessed 05/17/ 2019)

26. https://forum.lowcarber.org/showthread.php?t=50325 (Accessed 05/17/ 2019)

27. http://perfecthealthdiet.com/2012/02/the-trouble-with-pork-part-2/ (Accessed 05/18/ 2019)

28. http://www.nationalacademies.org/hmd/Reports/2002/Dietary-Reference-Intakes-for-Energy-Carbohydrate-Fiber-Fat-Fatty-Acids-Cholesterol-Protein-and-Amino-Acids.aspx. (Accessed 05/18/ 2019)

29. Westman EC, Phinney SD and Volek JS. The New Atkins for a New You: The Ultimate Diet for Shedding Weight and Feeling Great. A Touchstone Book, New York, London, Toronto, Sydney, New Delhi, 2010.

30. https://www.mayoclinic.org/healthy-lifestyle/nutrition-and-healthy-eating/in-depth/gout-diet/art-20048524 (Accessed 05/18/ 2019)

31. Holt SH, Brand-Miller JC, Petocz P. An insulin index of foods: the insulin demand generated by 1000-kJ portions of common foods. Am J Clin Nutr 1997; 66:1264–76.

32. Wright, JV. Dr. Wright's guide to healing with nutrition. Keats Publishing, Inc. New Canaan, Connecticut, 1984.

33. Freeman JM, Kossoff EH, Hartman AL (Mar 2007). The ketogenic diet: one decade later. Pediatrics. 119 (3): 535–43.

34. Grieb P, et al. Long-term consumption of a carbohydrate-restricted diet does not induce deleterious metabolic effects. Nutr Res.2008 Dec;28(12):825-33. doi: 10.1016/j.nutres.2008.09.011.

34. http://stan-heretic.blogspot.com/2010/ (Accessed 05/18/ 2019)

35. Johnson, H. Daintree; Love, A. H. G.; Rogers, N. C.; Wyatt, A. P.. Gastric ulcers, blood groups, and acid secretion. *Gut* , Oct1964, Vol. 5 Issue 5, p. 402-411, BMJ Publishing Group.

36. D'Adamo, J. The D'Adamo diet. Health Thru Herbs, Toronto, 1989.

37. Duke, JA. The Green pharmacy. Rodale Press, Emmaus, Pensylvania, 1997.

38. Kloss, J. Back to Eden. Back to Eden Books, Loma Linda, California, 1985.

39. Schiff L, Tahl T. The effects of dessicated hog's stomach in achlorhydria. Amer J Diges Dis, vol.1;1934-35:543-548.

40. https://link.springer.com/article/10.1007/BF03022442 (Accessed September 17, 2017)

41. http://coonplace.livejournal.com/59527.html (Accessed September 17, 2017)

42. https://www.youtube.com/watch?v=N9n6TlG4TeY (Accessed 07/10/2019)

43. Atkins, RC. Atkins for Life: The Complete Controlled Carb Program for Permanent Weight Loss and Good Health. St. Martin's

Press, New York, 2003.

44. Atkins, RC. Dr. Atkins' New Diet Revolution. Quill, An Imprint of HarperCollins Publishers, New York, 2002.

45. Maoshing Ni, Secrets of Longevity: Hundreds of Ways to Live to Be 100. Chronicle Books, San Francisco, 2006.

46. Paster, Z. with Meltsner, S. The Longevity Code: Your Personal Prescription for a Longer, Sweeter Life. Three rivers Press, New York, 2001.

47. Inlander, CB & Hodge, M. 100 Ways to Live to 100: The First Complete Guide to Living a Long and Productive Life. Wings Books, New York, Avenel, New Jersey, 1992.

48. Chopra, D. and Simon, D. Grow Younger: Ten Steps to Reverse Aging, Live Longer, Three rivers Press, New York, 2001.

49. Perls, TT., M.D. and Silver, MH., Ed.D. with Laurman, JF. Living to 100. Basic Books, New York, 1999.

50. Morris, MC. Diet for the Mind, Little, Brown and Company, New York, Boston, London, 2017.

51. Cantor, AJ. Dr. Cantor's Longevity Diet: How to Slow Down Aging and Prolong Youth and Vigor. Parker Publishing Company, Inc., West Nyack, N.Y., 1967.

52. Willcox BJ, Willcox DC and Suzuki, M. The Okinawa Program: How the World's Longest-Lived People Achieve Everlasting Health—and How You Can Too. Three rivers Press, New York, 2001.

53. Weil, A. Healthy Aging: A Lifelong Guide to Your Physical and Spiritual Well-Being. Alfred A. Knopf, New York, 2005.

54. Fulder, S. An End to Aging? Remedies for Life Extension. Destiny Books, New York, 1983.

55. Winick, M. Nutrition in Health and Disease. John Wiley & Sons, New York, 1980.

56. Bortz II, WM. We Live Too Short and Die Too Long:How to Achieve and Enjoy Your Natural 100-Year-Plus Life Span. Bantam Books, New York, Toronto, London, Sydney, Auckland, 1991.

57. Shealy, CN. Life Beyond 100: Secrets of the Fountain of Youth. Jeremy P. Tarcher/Penguin, New York, 2005.

58. Wallach, JD and Lan, M. Dead Doctors Don't Lie. Legacy Communications Group, Franklin, Tennessee, 1999.

59. Clement, B. Longevity: Enjoying Long Life without Limits. Jouvence Éditions, 2006.

60. Clement, B. Supplements Exposed: The Truth They Don't Want You to Know About Vitamins, Minerals, and Their Effects on Your Health. New Page Books, Franklin Lakes, N. J., 2010.

61. Li H, Fan YW, Li J, Tang L, Hu JN, Deng ZY. Evaluating and predicting the oxidative stability of vegetable oils with different fatty acid compositions. J Food Sci. 2013 Apr; 78(4): H633-41.

62. McCance, KL and Huether, SE. Pathophysiology: The Biologic Basis for Disease in Adults and Children. 4th ed., Mosby, Inc., St. Louis, Missouri, 2002.

63. Ayala, V., et al. Endogenous toxins associated with life expectancy and aging. In: Endogenous Toxins: Diet, Genetics, Disease and Treatment, O'Brien, PJ, Editor, WILEY-VCH Verlag, GmbH & Co., Weinheim, 2010, 769-786.

64. Arakawa K and Sagai M, Species differences in lipid peroxide levels in lung tissue and investigation of their determining factors. Lipids 21:769–765 (1986).

65. Taubes, G. Why We Get Fat and What to Do About It. Anchor Books, New York, 2011.

66. Yun J-M, and Surh J. Fatty Acid Composition as a Predictor for the Oxidation Stability of Korean Vegetable Oils with or without Induced Oxidative Stress. Prev Nutr Food Sci. 2012 Jun; 17(2): 158-165.

67. Pearson D, and Shaw S. Life Extension: A Practical Scientific Approach. Warner Books, Inc., New York, 1982.

68. http://nutritiondata.self.com/facts/fats-and-oils/507/2. (Accessed 05/18/ 2019). National Nutrient Database for Standard Refer., Release 26. United States Department of Agriculture, Agricultural Research Service.

69. http://nutritiondata.self.com/facts/fats-and-oils/621/2 (Accessed 05/18/ 2019)

70. Thompson, L.U. et al. Flaxseed and its lignan and oil components reduce mammary tumor growth at a late stage of carcinogenesis. Carcinogenesis, 1996,17(6):1373.

71. Delmonteque, R. Lifelong Fitness 2004. Longevity Publications, 2004.

72. Banaś, A. et al. Lipids in grain tissues of oat (Avena sativa): differences in content, time of deposition, and fatty acid composition. Journal of Experimental Botany, 2007, vol. 58, issue 10, 2463-70.

73. Bulgakov, M. Heart of the Dog (Sobachye Serdtse), a Russian novel.
https://www.goodreads.com/book/show/113205.Heart_of_a_Dog (Accessed 05/19/ 2019)

74. http://raypeat.com/articles/articles/unsaturated-oils.shtml (Accessed 05/19/ 2019)

75. Chopra, D, MD. Ageless Body, Timeless Mind: The Quantum Alternative to Growing Old. Harmony Books, New York, 1993.

76. http://whale.to/a/great_cholesterol_myth.html (Accessed 03/19/2018)

77. Schatz IJ1, Masaki K, Yano K, Chen R, Rodriguez BL, Curb JD. Cholesterol and all-cause mortality in elderly people from the Honolulu Heart Program: a cohort study. Lancet. 2001 Aug 4; 358(9279): 351-5.

78. Nago N, Ishikawa S, Goto T, Kayaba K: Low cholesterol is associated with mortality from stroke, heart disease, and cancer: the Jichi Medical School Cohort Study. J Epidemiol 2011;21:67–74.

79. Petursson H, Sigurdsson JA, Bengtsson C, Nilsen TI, Getz L: Is the use of cholesterol in mortality risk algorithms in clinical guidelines valid? Ten years prospective data from the Norwegian HUNT 2 study. J Eval Clin Pract 2012;18:159–168.

80. Weverling-Rijnsburger AW,Blauw GJ, Lag aay AM, Knook DL, Meinders AE, Westendorp RG: Total cholesterol and risk of mortality in the oldest old. Lancet 1997;350:1119–1123.

81. Neaton D, Blackburn H, Jacobs D. Serum cholesterol level mortality findings for men screened in the Multiple Risk Factor Intervention Trial. Multiple Risk Factor Intervention Trial Research Group, August 1992, Archives of Internal Medicine 152(7):1490-500.

82. Forette B, Tortrat D, Wolmark Y. Cholesterol as risk factor for mortality in elderly women. Lancet. 1989 Apr 22; 1 (8643): 868-70.

83. http://www.answers.com/Q/
What_does_threescore_and_ten_mean_in_the_Bible (Accessed 05/19/ 2019)

84. https://groups.google.com/forum/?hl=fi#!topic/sci.life-extension/zleU2SL7uIk (Accessed 05/19/ 2019)

https://www.youtube.com/watch?v=ZQsvYTHTudA (Accessed 05/19/ 2019)

85. Allard JP, Kurian R, Aghdassi E, Muggli R, Royall D. Lipid peroxidation during n-3 fatty acid and vitamin E supplementation in humans. Lipids. May 1997; 32(5): 535-541.

86. https://www.facebook.com/notes/brian-souter/macular-degeneration-do-vegetable-oils-cause-this-form-of-blindness/855550974493501/ (Accessed 05/19/ 2019)

87. http://www.sdadefend.com/Health/Canola-Hist.htm (Accessed 05/19/ 2019)

88. http://brincksm.weebly.com/uploads/3/6/3/4/3634133/communication_ar tifact.pdf (Accessed 05/19/ 2019)

89. http://www.fao.org/3/w3647e/W3647E07.htm (Accessed 05/19/ 2019)

90. Field CJ, Angel A, and Clandinin MT. Relationship of diet to the fatty acid composition of human adipose tissue structural and stored lipids. Am. J. Clin. Nutr. 1985, 42:1206–1220.

91. Malcom GT, Bhattacharyya AK, Velez-Duran M, Guzman MA, Oalmann MC, and Strong JP. Fatty acid composition of adipose tissue in humans: differences between subcutaneous sites. Am. J. Clin. Nutr., 1989, 50: 288–291.

92. Pamplona R. Membrane phospholipids, lipoxidative damage and molecular integrity: A causal role in aging and longevity. Biochimica et Biophysica Acta, September 2008, 1777(10):1249-62.

93. Guyenet SJ and Carlson SE. Increase in Adipose Tissue Linoleic Acid of US Adults in the Last Half Century. Adv Nutr November 2015 Adv Nutr vol. 6: 660-664, 2015.

94. Yam D, Eliraz A, Berry EM. Diet and disease–the Israeli paradox: possible dangers of a high omega-6 polyunsaturated fatty acid diet. Isr J Med Sci. 1996 Nov;32(11):1134-43.

95. Wolk A, Bergström R, Hunter D, Willett W, Ljung H, Holmberg L, Bergkvist L, Bruce A, Adami HO. A prospective study of association of monounsaturated fat and other types of fat with risk of breast cancer.

Arch Intern Med. 1998 Jan 12;158(1):41-5.

96. Mackie BS, Mackie LE, Curtin LD, Bourne DJ. Melanoma and dietary lipids. Nutr Cancer. 1987;9(4):219-26.

97. Fife, B. The Coconut Oil Miracle. 5th ed. Avery, New York, 2013.

98. Verburgh, K. The Longevity Code: Secrets of Living Well for Longer from the Front Lines of Science. The Experiment, LLC. New York, 2018.

99. Menotti A, et al. Food intake patterns and 25-year mortality from coronary heart disease: cross-cultural correlations in the Seven Countries Study. The Seven Countries Study Research Group." European Journal of Epidemiology 15, no. 6 (July 1999): 507-15.

100. Shanahan K with Shanahan L. Deep Nutrition: Why Your Genes Need Traditional Food. Flatoron Books, New York, 2008.

101. Grúz P, Shimizu M, et al. Mutagenicity of polyunsaturated fatty acid peroxidation products in the standard Ames assay.
http://www.nihs.go.jp/dgm/dgm2/ACN2015.pdf (Accessed 05/21/2019)

102. Brasky TM, Darke AK, ey al. Plasma phospholipid fatty acids and prostate cancer risk in the SELECT trial. J Natl Cancer Inst, 2013,105: 1132-1141.

103. Giovannucci E, Liu Y, Platz EA, Stampfer MJ, Willett WC. Risk factors for prostate cancer incidence and progression in the health professionals follow-up study. Int J Cancer. 2007,121: 1571-1578.

104. Sasaki T, Kobayashi Y, et al. Effects of dietary n-3-to-n-6 polyunsaturated fatty acid ratio on mammary carcinogenesis in rats. Nutr Cancer. 1998, 30: 137-143.

105. Olivo SE, Hilakivi-Clarke L Opposing effects of prepubertal low- and high-fat n-3 polyunsaturated fatty acid diets on rat mammary tumorigenesis. Carcinogenesis, 2005, 26: 1563- 1572.

106. https://budwigcenter.com/our-blog/budwig-protocol/ (Accessed 05/21/2019)

107. Frenkel EN, Neff WE, Bessier TR. Analysis of autoxidized fats by gas chromatography-mass spectrometry: V. Photosensitized oxidation. Lipids 1979, 14, 961.

108. Abdelhamid AS, Brown TJ, et. al., Omega-3 fatty acids for the primary and secondary prevention of cardiovascular disease. Cochrane Database of Systematic Reviews 2018, Issue 7. Art. No.: CD003177. DOI: 10.1002/14651858.CD003177.pub3.

https://www.ncbi.nlm.nih.gov/pubmed/30019766 (Accessed 05/22/2019)

109. https://health.gov/dietaryguidelines/2015/resources/DGA_Cut-Down-On-Saturated-Fats.pdf (Accessed 05/19/ 2019)

110. https://www.heart.org/en/healthy-living/healthy-eating/eat-smart/fats/polyunsaturated-fats (Accessed 05/19/ 2019)

111. Willett, WC., with Skerrett, PJ. Eat, Drink, and Be Healthy: The Harvard Medical School Guide to Healthy Eating. Free Press, New York, 2001.

112. Dawber, TR. Unproved Hypotheses. New England Journal of Medicine, 1978, 299, no. 9: 452-58.

113. https://www.accessdata.fda.gov/scripts/ InteractiveNutritionFactsLabel/ factsheets/ Monounsaturated_and_Polyunsaturated_Fat.pdf (Accessed 11/14/2019)

114. Purdin, H. Analytische Methoden zur Beurteilung der Frische und Haltbarkeit tierischer Fette, Fette Seifen Anstrichm. 77, 1976.

115. Weil, A., M.D. Eating Well for Optimal Health: The Essential Guide to Bringing Health and Pleasure Back to Eating, Quill, an Imprint of Harper Collins Publishers, 2001.

116. Frayn, KN. Metabolic Regulation: A Human Perspective. Portland Press, London, 1999.

117. Roediger WE. Role of anaerobic bacteria in the metabolic welfare of colonic mucosa in man. Gut. 1980; 21: 793–8.

118. https://www.nytimes.com/2013/10/09/dining/making-cultured-butter-at-home.html (Accessed 05/19/ 2019)

119. https://wholefoodcatalog.info/nutrient/butyric_acid/foods/high/ (Accessed 05/19/2019)

120. Smith JG, Yokoyama WH, German JB. Butyric acid from the diet: actions at the level of gene expression. Crit Rev Food Sci Nutr. 1998 May;38(4):259-97.

121. German JB. Butyric acid: a role in cancer prevention. Nutr Bull.

1999;24: 293-9.

122. Tang Y, Chen Y, Jiang H, Robbins GT, Nie D. G-protein-coupled receptor for short-chain fatty acids suppresses colon cancer. Int J Cancer. 2011 Feb 15;128(4):847-56.

123. Lad, V. Ayurveda: The Science of Self-healing. Lotus Press, Wilmot, WI, 1990.

124. Di Sabatino, A. et al. Oral butyrate for mildly to moderately active Crohn's disease. Aliment Pharmacol Ther. 2005 Nov 1;22(9):789-94.

125. Pituch A, Walkowiak J, Banaszkiewicz A Butyric acid in functional constipation. Prz Gastroenterol. 2013;8(5):295-8.

126. Balch, JF and Balch, PA. Prescription for Nutritional Healing. 2nd ed., New York: Avery Publishing Group, Inc., 1997.

127. McOrist AL, et al. Fecal butyrate levels vary widely among individuals but are usually increased by a diet high in resistant starch. J Nutr. 2011 May;141(5):883-9.

128. Banasiewicz T, Kaczmarek E, Maik J, et al. The influence of protected sodium butyrate on frequency and severity some clinical symptoms at the patients with irritable bowel syndrome. Gastroenterol Prakt. 2012;1:16–23.

129. Remely M., et al. Effects of short chain fatty acid producing bacteria on epigenetic regulation of FFAR3 in type 2 diabetes and obesity. Gene. 2014 Mar 1;537(1):85-92.

130. Gao Z, et al. Butyrate improves insulin sensitivity and increases energy expenditure in mice. Diabetes, 2009 Jul; 58(7):1509-17.

131. https://en.wikipedia.org/wiki/Michel_Eugène_Chevreul (Accessed 12/14/2019)

132. https://draxe.com/butyric-acid/ (Accessed 05/19/2019)

133. Teicholz, N. The Big Fat Surprise: Why Butter, Meat & Cheese Belong in a Healthy Diet. Simon & Schuster Paperbacks, New York, 2014.

134. Pinckney, ER and Pinckney, C. The Cholesterol Controversy. Sherbourne Press, Los Angeles, 1973.

135. Smith, RL. The Cholesterol Conspiracy. Warren H. Green, Inc., St. Louis, Missouri, 1991.

136. Constant, J. Nutritional management of diet-induced of

hyperlipidemias and atherosclerosis. Part II. Internal Medicine, 1987, 8, 145.

137. West, CE & Redgrave, TG. Reservations on the use of polyunsaturated fats in human nutrition. Search, 1974, 5. 90.

138. Kendrick, M. The Great Cholesterol Con: The Truth about What Really Causes Heart Disease and How to Avoid It. John Blake Publishing, London, 2007.

139. Leosdottir, M., et al. Dietary fat intake and early mortality patterns – data from The Malmo Diet and Cancer Study. J Intern Med, August 2005; 258(2), 153-65.

140. Rogers, SA. The Cholesterol Hoax. Sand Key Company, Inc., Sarasota, FL, 2008.

141. Taubes, G. Good Calories, Bad Calories: Challenging the Conventional Wisdom on Diet, Weight Control, and Disease. Alfred A. Knopf, New York, 2007.

142. Frantz ID, Jr., Dawson EA, Ashman PL, et al. Test of Effect of Lipid Lowering by Diet on Cardiovascular Risk. Arterioscler Thromb Vasc Biol. 1989;9:129-135.

143. Zamora D, Leelarthaepin B, et al. Use of dietary linoleic acid for secondary prevention of coronary heart disease and death: evaluation of recovered data from the Sydney Diet Heart Study and updated meta-analysis. BMJ 2013;346:e8707.

144. Rose GA, Thomson WB, Williams RT. Corn oil in treatment of ischaemic heart disease. BMJ, 1965;1:1531-3.

145. https://nutritiondata.self.com/facts/fats-and-oils/509/2 (Accessed 05/19/2019)

146. https://nutritiondata.self.com/facts/fats-and-oils/580/2 (Accessed 05/19/2019)

147. https://www.health.harvard.edu/staying-healthy/coconut-oil (Accessed 05/22/2019)

148. https://drhyman.com/blog/2016/04/06/is-coconut-oil-bad-for-your-cholesterol/ (Accessed 05/22/2019)

149. Barzilai N1, Atzmon G, et al. Unique lipoprotein phenotype and genotype associated with exceptional longevity. JAMA. 2003 Oct 15;290(15):2030-40.

150. Stipp, D. The Youth Pill: Scientists at the Brink of an Anti-Aging Revolution. Current, New York, 2010.

151. Lima TM, Kanunfre CC., et al. Ranking the toxicity of fatty acids on Jurkat and Raji cells by flow cytometric analysis. Toxicology in Vitro, 2002, 741-747.

152. Lokesh, B. R., S. N. Mathur, and A. A. Spector. Effect of fatty acid saturation on NADPH-dependent lipid peroxidation in rat liver microsomes. J. Lipid Res.1981;22: 905-915.

153. https://althealthworks.com/3477/video-how-this-man-reversed-his-als-lou-gehrigs-disease-symptoms-by-using-coconut-oil/ (Accessed 05/20/2019)

154. Law K, Azman N, et al. The effects of virgin coconut oil (VCO) as supplementation on quality of life (QOL) among breast cancer patients. Lipids Health Dis. 2014 Aug 27;13:139.

155. https://www.verywellhealth.com/caprylic-acid-89017 (Accessed 05/22/2019)

156. Kabara. J.J., Vrable, R. and Lie Ken Jie, M.S.F Antimicrobial Lipids: Natural and Synthetic Fatty Acids and Monoglycerides. Lipids, 1977;12:753-759.

157. Martin, MA, et al. Fatty acid composition in the mature milk of Bolivian forager-horticulturalists: controlled comparisons with a US sample. Matern Child Nutr. 2012 Jul; 8(3): 10.1111.

158. https://articles.mercola.com/sites/articles/archive/2009/09/22/7-reasons-to-eat-more-saturated-fat.aspx (Accessed 12/14/2019)

159. Kelly F, Sinclair AJ, et al. A stearic acid-rich diet improves thrombogenic and atherogenic risk factor profiles in healthy males. European Journal of Clinical Nutrition, March 2001;55(2):88-96.

160. Jick H, Slone D, Westerholm B, et al. Venous thromboembolic disease and ABO blood type: a cooperative study. Lancet. 1969;1:539–542.

161. Larsen TB, Johnsen SP, Gislum M, et al. ABO blood groups and risk of venous thromboembolism during pregnancy and the puerperium: a population-based, nested case-control study. J Thromb Haemost. 2005;3:300–304.

162. O'Donnell J, Laffan MA. The relationship between ABO histo-blood group, factor VIII and von Willebrand factor. Transfus Med. 2001; 11:343–351.

163. WHO Technical Report Series 916 Diet, Nutrition and the Prevention of Chronic Diseases, Report of a Joint WHO/FAO Expert Consultation, Geneva, 2003.

164. Pascual, G, et al. Targeting metastasis-initiating cells through the fatty acid receptor CD36. Nature, 2016, 10.1038/nature20791.

165. Watson, AL. Cereal Killer: The Unwanted Consequences of the Low Fat Diet. Diet Heart Publishing, Minneapoli, MN, 2009.

166. https://raypeatforum.com/community/threads/saturated-fats-and☐ mitochondrias.9177/ (Accessed 05/22/2019)

167. Lands, WEM. Historical perspectives on the impact of n-3 and n-6 nutrients on health. Progress in Lipid Research. July 2014;Vol 55, 17-29.

https://www.bmj.com/content/346/bmj.e8707 (Accessed 05/22/2019)

168. Gonzalez MJ., et al. Effect of dietary fat on growth of MCF-7 and MDA-MB231 human breast carcinomas in athymic nude mice: relationship between carcinoma growth and lipid peroxidation product levels. Carcinogenesis. 1991 Jul;12(7):1231-5.

169. Leaf, C. Think & Eat Yourself Smart: A Neuroscientific Approach to a Sharper Mind and Healthier Life. Baker Books, Grand Rapids, Michigan, 2016.

170. Dhaka, V., Gulia, N., Ahlawat, K. and Khatkar, B. Trans fats – Sources, health risks and alternative approach – A review. Journal of Food Science and Technology, 2011;48:534-541.

171. Phillips, K., Ruggio, D. and Amanna, K. Optimization of Standard Gas Chromatographic Methodology for the Determination of trans Fat in Unlabeled Bakery Products. Food Analytical Methods. 2010, 3: 277-294.

172. Kummerow FA, et al. Trans fatty acids in hydrogenated fat inhibited the synthesis of the polyunsaturated fatty acids in the phospholipid of arterial cells. Life Sciences, April 2004;74, 22(16):2707-2723.

173. Mozaffarian, D., Cao, H., King, I. B., Lemaitre, R. N., Song, X., Siscovick, D. S. and Hotamisligil, G. S. Trans-Palmitoleic Acid,

Metabolic Risk Factors, and New-Onset Diabetes in U.S. Adults. Annals of Internal Medicine, 2010;153:790-799.

174. Tardy, A.L., Morio, B., Chardigny, J.M. and Malpuech Brugère, C. Ruminant and industrial sources of trans-fat and cardiovascular and diabetic diseases. Nutrition Research Reviews, 2011;24:111-117.

175. Kummerow, FA with Kummerow, JM. Cholesterol is Not the Culprit: A Guide to Preventing Heart Disease. Spacedoc Media, LLC, 2014.

176. Chen ZY, Pelletier G, Hollywood R, Ratnayake WMN. *Trans* fatty acid isomers in Canadian human milk. Lipids 1995;30:15-21.

177. Mozaffarian D, Katan MB, Ascherio A, Stampfer MJ, Willett WC. Trans fatty acids and cardiovascular disease. N Engl J Med. 2006;354(15):1601–1613.

178. https://en.wikipedia.org/wiki/Fred_Kummerow (Accessed 05/19/2019)

179. Johnston PV, Johnson OC, Kummerow FA. Occurrence of trans fatty acids in human tissue. Science126, 1957, 698–699.

180. Kummerow, FA. Cholesterol Won't Kill You But Trans Fat Could: Separating Scientific Fact from Nutritional Fiction. Not Avail, 2008.

181. Morris MC, Evans DA, Bienias JL, et al. Dietary fats and the risk of incident Alzheimer's disease. Arch Neurol 2003; 60:194-200.

182. Estruch R, Ros E, Salas-Salvadó J, Covas MI, Corella D, Arós F, Gómez-Gracia E, Ruiz-Gutiérrez V, Fiol M, Lapetra J, Lamuela-Raventos RM, Serra-Majem L, Pintó X, Basora J, Muñoz MA, Sorlí JV, Martínez JA, Martínez-González MA; PREDIMED Study Investigators. Primary prevention of cardiovascular disease with a Mediterranean diet [published correction appears in N Engl J Med. 2014;370:886]. N Engl J Med. 2013;368:1279–1290. doi: 10.1056/NEJMoa1200303.

183. Wang DD, Li Y, Chiuve SE, Stampfer MJ, Manson JE, Rimm EB, Willett WC, Hu FB. Association of specific dietary fats with total and cause-specific mortality. JAMA Intern Med. 2016;176:1134–1145.

184. https://web.archive.org/web/20110719200400/http://bloodcenter.stanford.edu/about_blood/blood_types.html (Accessed 05/19/2019)

185. Weissberg, SM. and Christiano, J. The Answer is in Your Blood type: Research Linking Your Blood Type and how it affects Your Life Span, Love and Compatibility, Your Likely Illness Profile, Diet and Exercise for Maximum Life. Personal Nutrition USA, Inc., Lake Mary, FL, 1999.

186. http://www.healthcareitnews.com/news/hospital-acquired-infections-state (Accessed 05/19/2019)

187. https://www.healthrevelations.com/2015/12/14/statins-weaken-immune-systems/ (Accessed 05/19/2019)

188. Li Y, Hruby A, Bernstein AM, Ley SH, Wang DD, Chiuve SE, Sampson L, Rexrode KM, Rimm EB, Willett WC, Hu FB. Saturated fats compared with unsaturated fats and sources of carbohydrates in relation to risk of coronary heart disease: a prospective cohort study. J Am Coll Cardiol. 2015;66:1538–1548.

189. Sacks FM, Lichtenstein AH, et al. Dietary Fats and Cardiovascular Disease. A Presidential Advisory From the American Heart Association. Circulation. 2017;135:00–00.

190. Holmes MD, Hunter DJ, Colditz GA, Stampfer MJ, Hankinson SE, Speizer FE, Rosner B, Willett WC. Association of dietary intake of fat and fatty acids with risk of breast cancer. JAMA. 1999 Mar 10;281(10):914-20.

191. http://www.who.int/news-room/feature-stories/detail/denmark-trans-fat-ban-pioneer-lessons-for-other-countries (Accessed 05/19/2019)

192. U.S. Food and Drug Administration. Food labeling: trans fatty acids in nutrition labeling, nutrient content claims, and health claims. 68, 2003, Federal Register 41433- 41506.

193. https://www.newscientist.com/article/dn10178-new-york-city-may-ban-hazardous-trans-fats/ (Accessed 05/19/2019)

194. Kummerow, F. Citizen Petition to ban partially hydrogenated fat from the American Diet. 21 CFR 1030 CitizenPetition.

195. https://www.nytimes.com/2015/06/17/health/fda-gives-food-industry-three-years-eliminate-trans-fats.html (Accessed 05/19/2019)

196. https://www.nytimes.com/2015/06/19/opinion/the-slow-death-of-trans-fats.html (Accessed 05/19/2019)

197. Health Canada: trans fat ban takes effect next year. CBC news, Sept. 15, 2016.

198. Martin, C. A., de Oliveira, C. C., Visentainer, J. V., Matsushita, M. and de Souza, N. E. Optimization of the selectivity of a cyanopropyl stationary phase for the gas chromatographic analysis of trans fatty acids. Journal of Chromatography, 2008, A 1194: 111-117.

199. https://nutritiondata.self.com/facts/fats-and-oils/7948/2 (Accessed 05/19/2019)

200. https://nutritiondata.self.com/facts/fats-and-oils/624/2 (Accessed 05/19/2019)

201. http://nutritiondata.self.com/facts/fats-and-oils/635/2 (Accessed 05/19/2019)

202. https://nutritiondata.self.com/facts/fats-and-oils/636/2 (Accessed 05/19/2019)

203. https://nutritiondata.self.com/facts/fats-and-oils/10038/2 (Accessed 05/19/2019)

204. https://nutritiondata.self.com/facts/fats-and-oils/7947/2 (Accessed 05/19/2019)

205. https://nutritiondata.self.com/facts/fats-and-oils/7946/2 (Accessed 05/19/2019)

206. https://nutritiondata.self.com/facts/fats-and-oils/9129/2 (Accessed 05/19/2019)

207. https://nutritiondata.self.com/facts/fats-and-oils/621/2 (Accessed 05/19/2019)

208. https://nutritiondata.self.com/facts/fats-and-oils/7577/2 (Accessed 05/19/2019)

209. O'Keefe S, Gaskins-Wright S, Wiley V & Chen IC (1994) Levels of trans geometrical isomers of essential fatty acids in some unhydrogenated U.S. vegetable oils. Journal of Food Lipids 1, 165-176.

210. Vermunt SHF, et al. Dietary trans—-linolenic acid from deodorised rapeseed oil and plasma lipids and lipoproteins in healthy men: the TransLinE Study. British Journal of Nutrition, 2001, 85, 387-392.

211. https://nutritionfacts.org/video/trans-fat-saturated-fat-and-cholesterol-tolerable-upper-intake-of-zero/ (Accessed 05/20/2019)

212. American Diabetes Association. Complete Guide to Diabetes. Alexandria, VA, 1997.

213. Ornish, D. Dr. Dean Ornish's Program for Reversing Heart

Disease. New York: Random House, 1990.

214. Torelli, J. with Ryan, G. Beyond Cholesterol: 7 Life-Saving Heart Disease Tests That Your Doctor May Not Give You. St. Martin's Griffin, New York, 2005.

215. https://ndb.nal.usda.gov/ndb/ (Accessed 05/20/2019)

216. http://www.neoda.org.uk/oils-fats-information (Accessed 05/20/2019)

217 [174]. http://nutritiondata.self.com/facts/fats-and-oils/508/2 (Accessed 05/20/2019)

218 [175]. http://nutritiondata.self.com/facts/fats-and-oils/575/2 (Accessed 05/20/2019)

219 [176]. http://nutritiondata.self.com/facts/dairy-and-egg-products/133/2 (Accessed 05/20/2019)

220 [177]. http://nutritiondata.self.com/facts/fats-and-oils/482/2 (Accessed 05/20/2019)

221 [178]. http://nutritiondata.self.com/facts/fats-and-oils/510/2 (Accessed 05/20/2019)

222 [179]. http://nutritiondata.self.com/facts/fats-and-oils/483/2 (Accessed 05/20/2019)

223 [180]. http://nutritiondata.self.com/facts/fats-and-oils/598/2 (Accessed 05/20/2019)

224 [181]. http://nutritiondata.self.com/facts/fats-and-oils/509/2 (Accessed 05/20/2019)

225 [182]. http://nutritiondata.self.com/facts/fats-and-oils/7947/2 (Accessed 05/20/2019)

226 [183]. https://nutritiondata.self.com/facts/fats-and-oils/580/2 (Accessed 05/20/2019)

227 [184]. http://nutritiondata.self.com/facts/fats-and-oils/507/2 (Accessed 05/20/2019)

228 [185]. http://nutritiondata.self.com/facts/fats-and-oils/628/2 (Accessed 05/20/2019)

229 [186]. Ramprasath VR, Eyal I, Zchut S, Jones PJ. Enhanced increase of omega-3 index in healthy individuals with response to 4-week n-3 fatty acid supplementation from krill oil versus fish oil. Lipids Health Dis. 2013;12:178. doi: 10.1186/1476-511X-12-178.

Ramprasath VR, Eyal I., et al. Supplementation of krill oil with high phospholipid content increases sum of EPA and DHA in erythrocytes compared with low phospholipid krill oil. Lipids in Health and Disease, 2015;14:142.

230. St-Onge M-P and Bosarge A. Weight-loss diet that includes consumption of medium-chain triacylglycerol oil leads to a greater rate of weight and fat mass loss than does olive oil. Am. J Clin Nutr. 2008 Mar;87(3):621-626.

231. Assunção ML1, Ferreira HS, et al. Effects of dietary coconut oil on the biochemical and anthropometric profiles of women presenting abdominal obesity. Lipids. 2009 Jul;44(7):593-601.

232. Khaw KT, Sharp SJ, et al. Randomized trial of coconut oil, olive oil or butter on blood lipids and other cardiovascular risk factors in healthy men and women. BMJ Open. 2018 Mar 6;8(3):e020167.

233. Harcombe, Z. The Obesity Epidemic: What caused it? How can we stop it? Columbus Publishing Ltd., UK, 2010.

234. Prior IA, Davidson F, Salmond CE, Czochanska Z. Cholesterol, coconuts, and diet on Polynesian atolls: a natural experiment: the Pukapuka and Tokelau island studies. Am J Clin Nutr, 1981, 34, 1552-1561.

235. Vijayakumar M, Vasudevan DM, Sundaram KR, et al. A randomized study of coconut oil versus sunflower oil on cardiovascular risk factors in patients with stable coronary heart disease. Indian Heart J, 2016;68:498–506.

236. https://www.nytimes.com/2006/10/10/health/nutrition/10cons.html (Accessed 05/20/2019)

237. https://www.webmd.com/diet/features/trans-fats-science-and-risks#2 (Accessed 05/20/2019)

238. Gayet-Boyer C, Tenenhaus-Aziza F, Prunet C, et al. Is there a linear relationship between the dose of ruminant *trans*-fatty acids and cardiovascular risk markers in healthy subjects: results from a systematic review and meta-regression of randomized clinical trials. The British Journal of Nutrition. 2014;112(12):1914-1922. doi:10.1017/S0007114514002578.

239. http://www.zoeharcombe.com/the-knowledge/fat-does-not-clog-up-our-arteries/ (Accessed 05/20/2019)

240. Feillet-Coudray C., Aoun M., Fouret G., Bonafos B., Ramos J., Casas F., Cristol J.P., Coudray C. Effects of long-term administration of saturated and n-3 fatty acid-rich diets on lipid utilization and oxidative stress in rat liver and muscle tissues. Br. J. Nutr. 2013;110:1789–1802. doi:10.1017/S0007114513001311.

241. Dintenfass, L., The Role of ABO blood groups in blood rheology of cardiovascular disorders. Angiology. Jul/Aug 1973;24(7): 422-453.

242. O'Donnell J, Laffan MA. The relationship between ABO histo-blood group, factor VIII and von Willebrand factor. Transfus Med. 2001;11:343–351.

243. Littauer, F. How to Understand Others by Understanding Yourself Personality Plus. New York, Fleming H. Revell Company, 1983.

244. https://learninghotspot.wordpress.com/2017/01/06/how-overindulgence-in-sex-is-destructive-and-how-to-get-rid-of-it/ (Accessed 05/20/2019)

245. https://www.stress.org/stress-and-heart-disease/ (Accessed 05/20/2019)

246. https://www.nejm.org/doi/full/10.1056/NEJMoa1404881 (Accessed 05/20/2019)

247. Gill SS, Tuteja N. Reactive oxygen species and antioxidant machinery in abiotic stress tolerance in crop plants. Plant Physiology and Biochemistry, 2010, 48: 909-930.

248. Davies, KJA. Oxidative stress, antioxidant defenses, and damage removal, repair, and replacement systems, IUBMB Life, 2001, 50: 279-289.

249. https://lipidlibrary.aocs.org/chemistry/physics/plant-lipid/the-oxylipin-biosynthetic-pathways-in-plants (Accessed 07/24/2019)

250. Long, E. K., Picklo, M. J., Trans-4-hydroxy-2-hexenal, a product of n-3 fatty acid peroxidation: Make some room HNE. Free Radic. Biol. Med. 2010, 49, 1-8.

251. Stewart RRC. and Bewley, D. Lipid Peroxidation Associated with Accelerated Aging of Soybean Axes'. Plant Physiol. 1980, 65: 245-248.

252. Spickett CM. The lipid peroxidation product 4-hydroxy-2-

nonenal: Advances in chemistry and analysis. Redox Biol. 2013;1:145–152.

253. http://mpoc.org.my/upload/Understanding-Oils-Fats-Processing☐ aspects-practice-KimJongGil-POTS-Korea-2015-P1.pdf (Accessed 05/20/2019)

254. Seppanen, CM and Csallany, AS. Formation of 4-hydroxynonenal, a toxic aldehyde, in soybean oil at frying temperature. Journal of the American Oil Chemists' Society. 2002;79(10):1033-1038. (Accessed 12/22/2019)

255. Fujioka, K and Shibamoto, T. Formation of genotoxic dicarbonyl compounds in dietary oils upon oxidation. Lipids, 2004 May; 39(5):481-6.

256. Jacobs AT., Marnett LJ. Systems analysis of protein modification and cellular responses induced by electrophile stress. Acc. Chem. Res. 2010;43:673–683. 10.1021/ar900286y

257. Little, RC and Little, WC. Physiology of the Heart and Circulation, 4th ed. Year Book Medical Publishers, Inc. Chicago, 1989.

258. Sinisalo, J., et al. Relation of inflammation to vascular function in patients with coronary heart disease. Atherosclerosis, 2000, 149(2):403.

259. Mamonov V. Control for Life Extension. A Personalized Holistic Approach. Long Life Press, Co. 2001.

260. Rubin, AL. Diabetes for Dummies. Hungry Minds, New York, 2001.

261. Fried LP, Kronmal RA et al. Risk factors for 5-year mortality in older adults: the Cardiovascular Health Study. JAMA. 1998 Feb 25;279(8):585-92.

262. Greger, M with Stone, G. How Not to Die, Flatiron Books, New York, Ebook edition.

263. Roberts WC. It's Cholesterol, Stupid! Am J Cardiol. 2010;106(9):1364-6.

264. https://people.com/archive/dr-george-mann-says-low-cholesterol-diets-are-useless-but-the-heart-mafia-disagrees-vol-11-no-3/

265. Mann GV, Spoerry A, Gray M and Jarashow D. Atherosclerosis in the Masai. Am J Epidemiol 95: 26–37, 1972.

266. Shibata H, Nagai H. et al. Nutrition for the Japanese elderly. Nutr Health. 1992;8(2-3):165-75.

267. http://www.cnn.com/COMMUNITY/transcripts/2000/5/30/atkins.ornish/

268. https://ninateicholz.com/critique-of-dean-ornish-op-ed/

269. https://nutritionfacts.org/video/dr-gundrys-the-plant-paradox-is-wrong/

270. https://nutritionfacts.org/video/blood-type-diet-debunked/

271. https://twitter.com/bigfatsurprise/status/949759252863901697?lang=en

272. Dyerberg J, Bang HO, Hjorne N. Fatty acid composition of the plasma lipids in Greenland Eskimos. Am J Clin Nutr.1975 Sep;28(9): 958-66.

273. Bjerregaard P, Young TK and Hegele RA. Low incidence of cardiovascular disease among the Inuit—what is the evidence? Atherosclerosis 166 (2003) 351-357.

274. https://www.latimes.com/archives/la-xpm-1985-07-04-vw-9280-story.html

275. https://theskepticalcardiologist.com/2015/08/04/the-incredibly-bad-science-behind-dr-esselstyns-plant-based-diet/

276. Beasley, DeAnna E et al. "The Evolution of Stomach Acidity and Its Relevance to the Human Microbiome." PloS one. Jul. 2015; 10,7 e0134116. 29 doi:10.1371/journal.pone.0134116.

277. http://www.zoeharcombe.com/2018/01/food-to-help-you-live-longer/

278. Barnard ND, Cohen J, Jenkins DJ, et al. A low-fat, vegan diet improves glycemic control and cardiovascular risk factors in a randomized clinical trial in individuals with type 2 diabetes. Diabetes Care 2006;29: 1777–83.

279. Barnard ND, Cohen J, et al. A low-fat vegan diet and a conventional diabetes diet in the treatment of type 2 diabetes: a randomized, controlled, 74-wk clinical trial1–4. Am J Clin Nutr 2009; 89 (suppl):1588S–96S.

280. King, GL with Flippin, R. The Diabetes Reset: Avoid It. Control It. Even Reverse It. A Doctor's Scientific Program. Workman Publishing, New York, 2014.

281. Hsu WC, Lau KHK, Matsumoto M, Moghazy D, Keenan H, King GL (2014) Improvement of Insulin Sensitivity by Isoenergy High Carbohydrate Traditional Asian Diet: A Randomized Controlled Pilot Feasibility Study. PLoS ONE 9(9): e106851. https://doi.org/10.1371/journal.pone.0106851

282. http://www.diabetes.org/diabetes-basics/myths/ (Accessed 08/06/2019)

283. Mercola, J. Fat for Fuel: A Revolutionary Diet to Combat Cancer, Boost Brain Power, and Increase Your Energy Hay House, Inc., Carlsbad, CA, 2017.

284. Shai I, R.D., Ph.D., Schwarzfuchs D, M.D., et. al. Weight Loss with a Low-Carbohydrate, Mediterranean, or Low-Fat Diet. N Engl J Med 2008.

285. Enzinger C, Fazekas F, et al. Risk factors for progression of brain atrophy in aging. Six-year follow-up of normal subjects. Neurology, May 24, 2005; 64 (10), 1704-11.

286. Ahrens EH, Hirsch J. et al. Carbohydrate-induced and fat-induced lipemia. Transactions of the Medical Society of London, 1961, 74: 134-46.

287. https://www.ncbi.nlm.nih.gov/pmc/articles/PMC3584645/ (Accessed 05/20/2019)

288. https://www.youtube.com/watch?v=gCIhUebuy4w

289. Frayn, KN. Metabolic Regulation: A Human Perspective. 3rd ed., Wiley-Blackweel, 2010.

290. https://nutritiondata.self.com/mynd/mytracking/tracking-analysis

291. Marques-Lopes I, et al. Postprandial de novo lipogenesis and metabolic changes induced by a high-carbohydrate, low-fat meal in lean and overweight men. Am J Clin Nutr. 2001 Feb;73(2):253-61.

292. https://archive.org/details/DietForANewAmerica

293. http://180degreehealth.com/ray-peat-%E2%80%93-protein-and-vegetarian-diets/ (Accessed Oct 27 2018).

294. Cholesterol confusion: Let's make sense of it. Good Medicine. From the Physicians Committee for Responsible Medicine, Spring 2015, vol. XXIV, No. 2.

295. https://themedicalbiochemistrypage.org/amino-acids.php (Accessed 05/22/2019)

296. https://www.sciencedirect.com/topics/biochemistry-genetics-and-molecular-biology/essential-amino-acids (Accessed 05/22/2019)

297. http://www.alternativehealthatlanta.com/wp/wp-content/uploads/2012/07/essential-amino-acids-in-plant-based-foods1.pdf (Accessed 05/22/2019)

298. https://greatist.com/health/complete-vegetarian-proteins (Accessed 05/22/2019)

299. https://www.sciencedirect.com/science/article/pii/S0960852409006476 (Accessed 05/22/2019)

300. https://www.sciencedirect.com/topics/medicine-and-dentistry/nitrogen-balance (Accessed 05/22/2019)

301. http://cebp.aacrjournals.org/content/cebp/24/1/32.full.pdf (Accessed 05/22/2019)

302. https://www.myfooddata.com/articles/high-phenylalanine-foods.php (Accessed 05/22/2019)

303. http://raypeat.com/articles/aging/tryptophan-serotonin-aging.shtml (Accessed 05/22/2019)

304. Segall PE, Timiras PS, Walton JR. Low tryptophan diets delay reproductive aging. Mech Ageing Dev 1983 Nov-Dec; 23(3-4):245-52.

305. Richie JP Jr, Leutzinger Y, Parthasarathy S, Malloy V, Orentreich N, Zimmerman JA. Methionine restriction increases blood glutathione and longevity in F344 rats. FASEB J 1994 Dec;8(15):1302-7.

306. Caro P1, Gómez J, López-Torres M, Sánchez I, Naudí A, Jove M, Pamplona R, Barja G. Forty percent and eighty percent methionine restriction decrease mitochondrial ROS generation and oxidative stress in rat liver. Biogerontology,2008 Jun;9(3):183-96. doi: 10.1007/s10522-008-9130-1. Epub 2008 Feb 19.

307. Ruiz MC1, Ayala V, Portero-Otín M, Requena JR, Barja G, Pamplona R. Protein methionine content and MDA-lysine adducts are inversely related to maximum life span in the heart of mammals. Mech Ageing Dev, 2005 Oct;126(10):1106-14.

308. https://raypeat.com/articles/articles/gelatin.shtml (Accessed 05/22/2019)

309. Acheson KJ: Influence of autonomic nervous system on nutrient-induced thermogenesis in humans. Nutrition. 1993;9(4):373-80.

310. Watson, R. Eggs and Health Promotion. Ames, Iowa: Iowa State Press, 2002.

311. http://www.naturelaws.org/engl/shatalova.html (Accessed 05/23/2019)

312. https://en.wikipedia.org/wiki/Teresa_Hsu (Accessed 05/23/2019)

313. https://deniseminger.com/for-vegans/ (Accessed 05/23/2019)

314. https://deniseminger.com/2016/10/20/why-do-some-people-do-well-as-vegans-and-vegetarians-clues-from-the-magical-world-of-genetics/ (Accessed 05/23/2019)

315. https://articles.mercola.com/sites/articles/archive/2014/09/03/too-much-protein.aspx (Accessed 05/23/2019)

316. https://academic.oup.com/jn/article/130/7/1868S/4686204 (Accessed 05/23/2019)

317. https://www.dietaryfiberfood.com/protein/protein-requirement-for-humans.php (Accessed 05/23/2019)

318. Diamond, H and M. Fit For Life. Warner Books, Inc., New York, 1985.

319. Rose, W. C. (1957) The amino acid requirements of adult man. Nutr. Abstr. Rev. 27: 631–647.

320. Hegsted, D. M. (1963) Variation in requirements of nutrientsamino acids. Fed. Proc. 22: 1424–1430.

321. http://www.kidneyurology.org/Library/Kidney_Health/Nutrition_Later_Chronic_Kidney_Disease_Adults.php((Accessed 05/23/2019)

322. Schmidt, JA, et al. Plasma concentrations and intakes of amino acids in male meat-eaters, fish-eaters, vegetarians and vegans: a cross-sectional analysis in the EPIC-Oxford cohort. Eur J Clin Nutr. 2016 Mar; 70(3): 306–312. Published online 2015 Sep 23.

https://www.ncbi.nlm.nih.gov/pubmed/26395436 (Accessed 05/23/2019)

323. Veldhorst MA, Westerterp-Plantenga MS, Westerterp KR. Gluconeogenesis and energy expenditure after a high protein, carbohydrate-free diet. Am J Clin Nutr. 2009 Sep;90(3):519-26.

324. https://www.amazon.com/Nutrition-Vegetarians-Agatha-Thrash/dp/0942658035 (Accessed 05/23/2019)

325. http://chetday.com/normanwalker.htm (Accessed 05/23/2019)

326. Nishizawa, T. et al. Some factors related to obesity in the Japanese Sumo Wrestler. American Journal of Clinical Nutrition, November 1976, 29(10):1167-74.

https://academic.oup.com/ajcn/article-abstract/29/10/1167/4617102? redirectedFrom=fulltext (Accessed 05/23/2019)

327. Moriguchi EH, Moriguchi Y, YamoriY. Impact of diet on the cardiovascular risk profile of Japanese immigrants living in Brazil: contributions of World Health Organization CARDIAC and MONALISA studies. Clin Exp Pharmacol Physiol. 2004 Dec;31 Suppl 2:S5-7.

328. Shibata H, Nagai H, Haga H, Yasumura S, Suzuki T, Suyama Y. Nutrition for the Japanese elderly. Nutr Health. 1992;8(2-3):165-75.

329. Vogel, A. The Nature Doctor. Keats Pub., New Canaan, Conn.: 1991.

330. https://www.nap.edu/catalog/371/diet-nutrition-and-cancer (Accessed 05/23/2019)

331. Kushi, M and Jack, A. The Cancer Prevention Diet. St. Martin's, New York, 1983.

332. https://www.omicsonline.org/proceedings/estimating-annual-number-of-deaths-from-outdoor-air-pollution-in-bangkok-thailand-32178.html (Accessed 05/23/2019)

333. https://www.researchgate.net/publication/47815535_Nutrition_Transition_and_Cardiovascular_Disease_Risk_Factors_in_Middle_East_and_North_Africa_Countries_Reviewing_the_Evidence (Accessed 05/23/2019)

334. https://www.canceractive.com/article/the-role-of-gut-bacteria-in-colorectal-cancer-1342 (Accessed 05/23/2019)

Index

A

aging
  accelerated, 37
  anti-aging, 44
  brain, 68
Ahrens, Jr., Edward H., 106, 110
alcohol, 12, 36, 69, 89, 131
aldehydes, 44, 46, 89, 91, 125, 128,
  130
almonds, 21, 89
Alzheimer's disease, 39, 43, 57, 67–
  68, 128
American Heart Association AHA,
  33, 43, 47–48, 71
amino acids, 34, 42, 61, 94, 105–
  106, 108, 111–114, 116, 118–
  119, 126, 128, 130
ammonia, 114, 128
animal fat, 10, 13, 15, 17–18, 28–29,
  33, 35–39, 41, 48, 54–56, 63, 68,
  73, 86, 97, 109, 126, 130, 134
anti-nutrients, 8, 112, 128
apoptosis, 44, 57, 129
apples, 113, 119
arteriosclerosis, 129
arthritis, 6, 9–10, 12, 43, 58, 129,
  134
atherosclerosis, 19, 33, 57, 66, 92,
  97–100, 109, 129, 131
Atkins, Robert C., 10, 13–14, 98,
  103–104
avocados, 43, 99

Ayurveda, 3, 34, 49, 129

B

bacon, 13–15
Balch, James E., 50
Balch, Phyllis A., 50
bananas, 49, 51
Barnard, Neal, 110
beans
  navy, 29
  pinto, 29
  soy, 8
beef, 8–10, 13–14, 19, 28–29, 33,
  56, 59, 62–63, 67, 89, 107,
  113, 125–126
beets, 21, 93
bile, 20, 129
biochemistry, 62, 129
Blood type A1 diet, 5, 7, 9–12, 16,
  21, 29, 62, 126
blood types, 59, 63, 70, 86, 126
"blue zones," 93, 129
body constitution, 117, 129
body fat, 51, 133
body temperature, 31
bone broth, 10, 113, 126
bones, 2–3, 111, 131
Bortz II, Walter M., 20
bread
  white, 5, 15, 17, 29–30, 91, 93,
  106–107, 132
  whole-grain, 87

broccoli, 112
brown rice, 29, 112
Buerger's disease, 9
butyric acid, 48–51, 82, 129

C

cabbage, 6, 113
calcium, 10, 45, 79, 128–129, 134
calories, 3, 16, 18, 47, 54, 73, 103, 108, 110, 119, 121
Campbell, T. Colin, 109–110
cancer
    breast, 40, 45, 58–59, 61, 63, 65, 73, 112, 114, 122
    colon, 49–51, 122–124
    excessive protein intake and, 122-123
    gastric, 53
    kidneys, 19, 114, 122, 130
    pancreas, 10, 36, 94, 122, 130
    prostate, 45, 122
    rectum, 122
Cantor, Alfred J., 16–17
capillaries, 95
carbohydrates
    complex, 3–4, 62, 93, 109, 111, 119
    simple (refined), 93
carbon dioxide, 4, 93, 95, 114, 133, 135
cardiovascular disease
    deaths, 35, 46, 52, 55, 71–72, 74, 87, 95
    events, 46, 55, 68, 74, 87
    mortality, 34–36, 40, 43, 46, 53–55, 69, 72, 79, 95, 98
    risk, 11, 21, 23, 34–36, 40, 42–43, 45–47, 53, 57, 59–60, 66–67, 73, 79, 83, 87, 95–96, 105, 110, 122–123, 126, 130–131
cellular self-digestion, 58
centenarians, 15, 17, 97, 121, 127
cereals, 21, 30, 64, 71, 93, 133
Chaitow, Leon, 2
cheese, 8, 10, 15–16, 21, 28, 45, 52, 68, 107–108, 113, 120
chia, 30, 44, 88, 112
chickens, 8–9, 11, 115
chocolate, 67
cholesterol
    dietary, 9, 18–19, 40–41, 47, 49–50, 54–55, 60–62, 67–68, 70–71, 73, 91, 98–99, 103, 107, 110, 113–114, 117–119, 129–130, 135
    HDL, 57, 64, 79, 83, 87, 95
    LDL, 14, 47, 50, 57, 60, 63–64, 66, 78–79, 83, 95–96
    lowering, 20, 33, 55, 99, 126
    phobia of, 14, 34, 60
    theory of, 18
    war against, 18, 94
Chopra, Deepak, 15, 34
circulation, 129
Clement, Brian, 21–22, 29, 31, 103
Cochrane Collaboration, 46, 130
coffee, 11
colon, 49–51, 122–124
constipation, 51
copper, 90
corn, 8, 19, 32
coronary artery disease, 79, 98, 129, 131
C-reactive protein, 79, 83, 130
creatinine, 114, 130

Crohn's disease, 49–50, 59, 130
cysteine, 37, 105, 113, 126, 132

D

D'Adamo, Peter J., 50, 98
DASH study, 68
dates,
Delmoteque, Robert, 30
de novo lipogenesis, 61, 106, 108, 126, 130
dementia, 67–68, 130
depression, 37, 99
diabetes, 9–10, 21, 40, 51, 57–58, 69, 71, 74, 78, 84, 91, 95, 101–104, 110, 117, 120, 125–126, 130–131, 133
Diamond, Harvey, 118
Diamond, Marilyn, 118
diarrhea, 49, 51, 130
digestion, 11, 18, 49, 58, 93, 112, 119, 128–129
dill, 29

E

edema, 62, 130
epigenetic, 44, 131
estrogen, 131
exercise, 20, 99, 120, 129, 135

F

fasting
    dry, 4, 18
    glucose level, 95, 102, 105, 107–108, 130
    insulin, 10, 40, 79, 94–95, 106–108, 126, 130, 132
    water, 4, 31, 42, 61, 82, 84–85, 90, 93, 98, 114–115
fats
    animal, 2–3, 8–13, 15, 17–19, 22, 28–29, 33, 35–39, 41, 43–45, 48, 51, 54–56, 59, 61–63, 68, 70, 73, 84, 86, 97–98, 100–103, 109, 112–114, 119–122, 126, 129–131, 134
    peroxidized, 26, 33, 36, 128
    plant, 2–4, 14, 19, 22, 29, 44, 61–62, 71, 87–90, 93, 97–99, 109, 112–114, 116, 119, 126, 128–129, 132
    trans, 6, 14, 17, 26, 47, 60, 63–71, 73–77, 85–86, 90, 96, 102, 125
fatty acids
    essential, 2–4, 18–19, 21–22, 44, 93, 95, 97, 99, 101, 103, 111–112, 114, 116, 126, 132–133, 136
    long-chain, 45, 59, 82, 89, 134
    monounsaturated MUFA, 25
    omega-3, 24, 26–30, 42–46, 48, 61, 63, 69, 79, 98
    omega-6, 24, 26, 28, 40, 42, 44–45, 61, 63, 79, 131
    polyunsaturated PUFA, 5, 8, 13, 15–16, 19, 26, 30, 32–33, 37, 39–40, 48, 53–55, 61, 64, 73, 82, 89, 98, 102, 125, 132
    saturated SFA, 7, 12–16, 18–19, 21, 30, 33, 38–41, 43, 47–65, 67–68, 70–71, 73–74, 76, 78–79, 82–84, 86, 96–98, 100, 102, 115, 125, 129, 132, 134
    unsaturated USFA, 14, 16,

23, 32, 62, 73–74, 86

fish roe, 19

fitness, 30, 66, 97

Food and Drug Administration, 47, 66, 74–75

Framingham Heart Study, 131

Frayn, Keith, 107–108, 110

free radicals, 20, 23, 53, 89, 131–132, 134

French fries, 17, 90

French paradox, 54, 131

fried foods, 14, 17, 21, 31, 64, 66, 68

fruits, 15, 44, 56, 73, 93–94, 102, 112, 120

Fulder, Stephen, 18

G

garlic, 7, 50

gelatin, 113, 126, 131

ghee, 49, 51, 82, 131

ginger, 7, 11

ginseng, 11, 18

grains
    refined, 71, 93, 109
    whole, 2, 5, 10, 13, 15–16, 29–30, 34, 52, 54, 68–71, 87, 93, 100, 112–113

greens
    collard, 113
    dandelion, 49, 51
    mustard, 113

growth hormone, 131-132
    synthetic, 128

H

Harcombe, Zoë, 84

Health Professionals Follow-up HPFS Study, 45, 69–73, 86

heart disease, 19, 34–35, 41–43, 47, 52–55, 57–58, 65–66, 71, 74, 78, 84, 86–87, 96–100, 117, 120, 125–126, 131
    ischemic, 55
    latitude and, 88
    risk of, 11, 35–36, 40, 42–43, 47, 57, 60, 66–67, 73, 79, 110, 122, 126
    saturated fat and, 18–19, 54, 68, 83
    vegetable oils and, 18, 87, 103

"heart-healthy," 37, 41, 46, 48, 82–83

hemp seeds, 29, 82

hepatitis, 10, 12, 131

Hippocrates, 2

Hodge, Marie, 14

Holford, Patrick, 118

homocysteine, 79, 130, 132

honey, 1, 8, 93

hypertension, 40, 57, 68–69, 120

I

immune system
    inflammation and, 39, 83
    infections and, 82

indigestion, 11, 116

insulin, 10, 40, 79, 94-95, 106-108, 126, 130, 132
    hyperinsulinemia, 40
    resistance, 40, 49–50, 74, 95, 108, 130
    score, 27, 29, 31, 36, 63, 94

interleukin, 58, 132

iron, 90, 128, 134

J

Japanese centenarians, 97, 121
juice
    digestive, 49, 100, 119
    green, 31

K

ketogenic diet, 132
ketones, 132
Keys, Ancel, 43, 55, 69, 99–100
Klaper, Michael, 107–110
Kummerow, Fred A., 66–67, 74–75, 114
Kushi, Michio, 122
Kwasniewski, Jan, 9–10, 13, 103

L

LaLanne, Jack, 30
lamb, 8–9, 113
Lan, Ma, 21
lard, 9, 13–14, 16, 28, 37–39, 47, 52, 59, 62, 68
large intestine, 49
lauric acid, 59, 79, 82, 132
Leaf, Caroline, 64
lectins, 5–8, 98, 112, 128, 132
legumes, 6, 21, 44, 68, 93, 98, 102, 133
lentils, 6, 112–113
lifestyle, 11, 44, 117, 120, 131
lipid peroxidation, 26, 33, 36, 128
liver
    cancer of, 36, 122
    disease, 12, 21
longevity, 1–2, 5, 14–16, 18, 20–

21, 31–32, 36–37, 42–43, 51, 66, 93, 99, 112, 120–121, 129, 132–133
Longevity Quotient LQ, 132
lungs, 61–62
Lyon Diet Heart Study, 71, 87
lysine, 105, 111, 132

M

macular degeneration, 37, 43, 132
malondialdehyde MDA, 26–27, 37, 44, 58, 90–91, 130, 132
margarine, 17–18, 21, 26, 52, 55, 64, 68, 71, 76, 87
McDougal, John A., 109–110
meat
    crab, 8
    muscle, 2–3, 100, 106, 111, 113, 119, 126, 129–130, 132, 135
    organ, 2, 15, 19, 63, 91, 111, 130, 134–135
    prepared, 16, 64, 85, 104
    processed, 6, 11, 21, 41, 56, 64, 74, 84, 108, 124
    red, 11, 15–17, 44, 68, 87, 95, 100–101, 107, 129
    smoked, 16
    stock, 10, 113, 126
meditation, 4
Mediterranean diet, 29, 68, 133
medium-chain triglycerides MCTs, 82, 133
metabolic syndrome, 133
metabolic waste, 133
metabolism, 6, 10, 12, 18, 58, 61, 89, 91, 93, 95, 106, 109, 112– 114, 119–120, 130, 132–133,

135

methionine, 42, 111, 113–114, 126, 132–133

milk

 breast, 59, 61, 65, 112, 114

 coconut, 7–9, 13–14, 16, 21, 29, 39, 41, 47–48, 56–59, 63, 67, 79, 82–86, 88, 125, 133

 skimmed, 16

 whole, 2, 5, 10, 13, 15–16, 29–30, 34, 52, 54, 68–71, 87, 93, 100, 112–113

mind, 1–2, 4, 15–16, 68, 101, 135

MIND diet, 68

minerals, 3–4, 10, 34, 37, 116

Minnesota Coronary Survey, 54

Morris, Martha C., 15–16, 67–69

myocardial infarction, 35, 69, 87, 133

N

Ni, Maoshing, 14

nitrogen balance, 2, 112, 133

Nurses' Health Study NHS, 69–74, 86

nuts, 6–7, 10, 14–15, 21, 28, 30, 43–44, 48, 68, 87–91, 112–113, 120, 133

O

oats, 29–30, 44

obesity, 9, 40, 83–84, 120, 133

oil

 almond, 7, 14, 21, 25, 89

 borage, 21, 31

 camellia, 25, 27

 canola (rapeseed), 14, 26

 coconut, 7–9, 13–14, 16, 21, 29, 39, 41, 47–48, 56–59, 63, 67, 79, 82–86, 88, 125, 133

 cod liver, 15, 31–32, 54, 91

 cooking, 14–15, 17, 21, 26, 38, 41, 45–46, 52, 84–85, 90–91, 94, 101, 116, 126, 131

 corn, 13, 16, 38, 45, 55-56, 63, 91, 110

 cottonseed, 15, 32, 37–38

 deodorized, 76–77

 evening primrose, 29, 82

 fish, 14, 17, 22, 28, 31, 43, 60-61, 63-65, 69, 90

 flaxseed, 13, 29, 43, 48, 69

 grape seed, 13–14, 16, 26, 29, 82

 hemp seed, 25–26, 32, 112

 hydrogenated, 17, 26, 64, 68, 75–76, 86

 macadamia nut, 7–8, 29, 56, 67, 82

 olive, 13–16, 19, 26–27, 29–30, 37, 48, 55–56, 63, 68, 82–83, 87, 99, 133

 palm, 13, 25, 27, 48, 62, 86, 134

 palm kernel, 14, 48, 76, 82, 133

 partially hydrogenated, 75–76

 peanut, 7, 14, 21,

 perilla, 26–27

 peroxidized, 26, 33, 36, 128

 rancid, 5, 19, 22–23, 25, 29–31, 33, 36, 38, 42, 48, 56, 65, 82, 132

 safflower, 13–16, 19, 32, 37–38, 55, 82, 88

 salmon, 31, 42, 63, 88, 91

sesame, 14, 19, 25, 32
soybean, 9, 14–16, 25–26, 37–41, 48, 76, 82–83, 90–91, 112–113, 115
sunflower, 14–16, 19, 21, 25, 48, 56, 58, 82, 89
tropical, 14, 17, 39, 48, 84, 86, 88
tuna, 42, 91
walnut, 14, 21, 43, 48
olives, 43, 56
onions, 13
green, 21, 30–31, 49, 87
optimal nutrition, 9
Ornish, Dean, 97-99, 110
overweight, 71, 108, 114

P

pain
abdominal, 51, 83
joint, 49, 95, 129, 131, 134–135
palmitic acid, 59–62, 134
pancreas, 10, 36, 94, 122, 130
parsley, 29
Paster, Zorba, 14, 42
peanuts, 112
Pearson, Durk, 33–34, 60
Peat, Ray, 12, 32–33, 109, 113
Perlmutter, David, 68
Perls, Thomas T., 15
Peroxidability Index PI, 24–25, 27, 39–40, 79, 86, 134
phytic acid, 112, 128, 134
Pinckney, Cathey, 52
Pinckney, Edward R., 52
pizzas, 64
poison, 9, 32, 87

pork, 8–9, 16–17, 33, 97, 113
potatoes
sweet, 6, 9, 21, 39, 84
yams, 1, 6
poultry, 8, 15, 17, 33, 44, 87, 97, 112
processed foods, 6, 84
Progesterone, 134
Prolactin, 134
prostate, 45, 122
protein metabolism, 120, 135
proteins
animal, 2–3, 8–13, 15, 17–19, 22, 28–29, 33, 35–39, 41, 43–45, 48, 51, 54–56, 59, 61–63, 68, 70, 73, 84, 86, 97–98, 100–103, 109, 112–114, 119–122, 126, 129–131, 134
plant-based, 22, 44, 71, 97, 99, 109, 113–114, 126
plasma, 17, 37, 59, 77, 102, 106–108, 110
purines, 10, 134

Q

quinoa, 29–30, 44, 112

R

raw food diet, 115–116
reactive carbonyl compounds, 23, 134
reactive oxygen species ROS, 89, 113, 134
relationships, 2
rheumatoid arthritis, 10, 43, 134
Robbins, John, 109
ruminants, 8, 112, 134

S

salmon, 31, 42, 63, 88, 91
sauerkraut, 6
sausages, 32
science, 1, 46, 66, 99, 122, 129
    nutritional, 69
seaweed, 8
selenium, 37
semen, 134
sex, 87, 95, 130–131, 135
Shanahan, Katherine, 44–45
Shatalova, Galina, 115, 118
Shaw, Sandy, 33
Shealy, C. Norman, 20-21
sleep, 2
small intestine, 49–50, 108, 129
Smith, Russel L., 53
smoking, 45, 69, 87, 123, 130
snacks, 93
soy beans, 8
starches
    resistant, 39, 49, 51, 63
stress, 2, 18, 87, 100
    oxidative, 23, 39, 44, 48, 113,
    125, 131
stroke, 35, 47, 54, 78, 92, 98, 105,
    117, 125–126, 129, 131, 134
sumo wrestlers, 120–121, 135
sunlight, 2, 4
Suzuki, Makoto, 16
Sydney Diet Heart Study, 55

T

Taubes, Gary, 26
teeth, 111
Teicholz, Nina, 52, 98, 110
testosterone, 135

thiobarbituric acid, TBA, 63, 135
thyroid gland, 6, 58, 135
tofu, 17, 48
tomatoes, 6, 112
Torelli, Julius, 79
toxins, 8, 31, 61, 135
    endogenous, 31, 37, 91, 135
    environmental, 117
Traditional Chinese Medicine, 3,
    135
tumors, 44, 63, 129
    breast, 45
tuna, 42, 91
turkey, 8, 100

U

urea, 114, 135
uric acid, 134–135
urine, 114, 117–118, 133
USDA, 26, 28, 76, 79

V

vegetables
    cruciferous, 6
    root, 19, 87, 115
    sea, 84, 120
    starchy, 94
vegetarian diet, 109, 113
vegetarians, 119–120
Verburgh, Kris, 42–44, 46
vitality, 9, 135
vitamins
    multivitamins, 69
    vitamin C, 6
    vitamin D, 130
    vitamin E, 37, 63, 69
Vogel, A, 122

Index

W

Walker, Norman, 120
Wallach, Joel D., 21
walnuts, 21, 43
wastes, 2
weight loss, 26, 30, 49, 58, 82, 103, 114, 132, 135
Weil, Andrew, 17, 19
wheat, 8, 29
   grass, 29
Willcox, Bradley J., 16
Willcox, D. Craig, 16
Willett, Walter C., 47, 73
Winick, Myron, 18–19

women, 34–36, 40, 51–54, 58, 61, 70, 72–74, 83, 95, 100
World Health Organization WHO, 60, 74, 135
worry, 8, 36, 135
Wright, Jonathan V., 50

Y

Yamamoto, Shizuko, 2
yoga, 99, 136
yogurt, 10, 115

Z

zinc, 36, 134, 137

About the Author

Valery Mamonov, Ph. D., was born and educated in Russia, where he studied holistic methods and experimented with fasting, various diets, and alternative therapies for more than 20 years. He left his successful career as a consulting engineer in 1996 to concentrate full time on creating a program that would offer a new approach to health and longevity. In 2001 he published the book, "Control for Life Extension. A Personalized Holistic Approach," which was based on his research and interviews with centenarians and long-living people in the United States, Iceland, Singapore, Russia, and Japan.

He is living proof of the rightness of his ideas on health: his Blood type is A (subtype A1), members of which have the shortest life expectancy of all Blood types, only 62 years. Also, he is tall, 6'2", which works against him as well: six years must be subtracted from his life expectancy because of his height. Despite of his body constitutional disadvantages, at his age of 78 he is still going strong and is free of medications. His answer is in a diet and a lifestyle designed to suite his body type.

He had lived in Rome, Maine for 20 years and now lives in Fort Pierce, Florida.

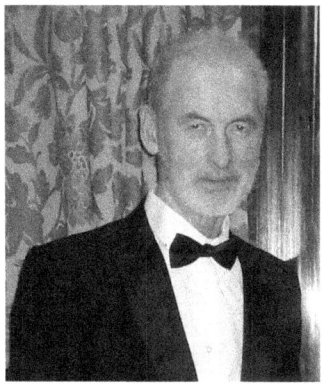

www.longevitywatch.com/index.html
valmamonov@holtmail.com

www.ingramcontent.com/pod-product-compliance
Lightning Source LLC
Chambersburg PA
CBHW060505290526
45791CB00001B/275